CRYSTAL
MESH

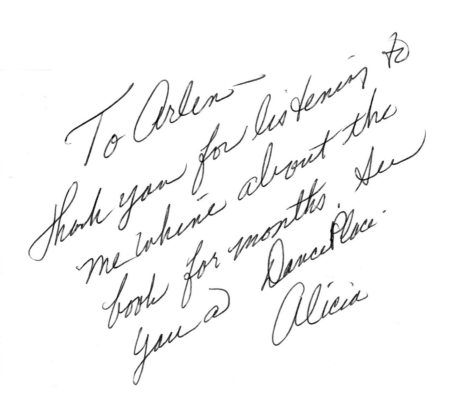

To Arlen—

Thank you for listening to me whine about the book for months. See you @ Dance Place.

Alicia

CRYSTAL MESH

How Addiction to Money Turned Medical Device Makers, the FDA, and Doctors Into Street Dealers

ALICIA MUNDY WITH JENNIFER BANMILLER

Published by Periscope Group, Danville, CA
www.periscopegroup.com

Cover Design: Blake Brysha
Image Credits: Mesh Images – Dionysios K. Veronikis, MD;
Diagrams – Wingtip Communications Inc.

ISBN (paperback): 978-1-7334315-0-7
e-ISBN: 978-1-7334315-1-4

First Edition

Printed in the United States of America

CONTENTS

FOREWORD vii

ACKNOWLEDGMENTS ix

IN THEIR OWN WORDS xv

INTRODUCTION 1

CHAPTER 1 5
CAPITALISM GONE WILD

CHAPTER 2 27
HOW THE DEAL WENT DOWN

CHAPTER 3 47
WALLET-DRIVEN MISSION

CHAPTER 4 69
PUSHERS

CHAPTER 5 95
DO NO F****** HARM!

CHAPTER 6 109
VA-CHING!

CHAPTER 7 131
KINGPINS IN THE EXECUTIVE OFFICE

CHAPTER 8 . . . . **141**
DOWN UNDER . . . THE SILENT RECALL

CHAPTER 9 . . . . **155**
BEST HIGH IN TOWN

CHAPTER 10 . . . . **175**
THE IRREGULAR REGULATORY PROCESS

CHAPTER 11 . . . . **197**
DEMIGODS

CHAPTER 12 . . . . **217**
THE HONEY POT

CHAPTER 13 . . . . **233**
SLINGS AND ARROWS

CHAPTER 14 . . . . **245**
BREAKING BAD

CHAPTER 15 . . . . **267**
MESHED UP

CHAPTER 16 . . . . **289**
REDEMPTION—A WINNING PROPOSITION

TVM TIMELINE OF DESTRUCTION **311**

SOURCES **315**

ABOUT THE AUTHORS **335**

FOREWORD

For 25 years, my company has given consumers help connecting to credible legal access in an overcrowded industry that is hard to navigate. For the most part, it has been a truly inspirational journey working with professionals in this legal and medical field who are fighting for people for the right reasons.

As a consumer marketing company, we have worked on almost every warning, recall, and off-label catastrophe over the last two decades, starting with asbestos and fen-phen in 1994. For the past seven years, we have been front row to everything mesh: the women and their stories, the carnage, the pleas for help, and the litigation that ensued because of greed. Mesh has been one of the most catastrophic of all products or drugs sold on the market.

To the hundreds of thousands of women who have called us over the years and trusted us with the stories of your lives, your experiences with the legal and medical world, and the carnage to your bodies because of mesh, please accept my most sincere thank-you. You do have a voice, and you have been unforgettably heard.

And to Carmen, who has always encouraged me to do the right thing, even if it wasn't the most popular thing. Writing this book has been eye opening and certainly not popular. We were told many times to "stay in our lane" and to not rock the boat on mesh. Lawyers, medical device sales representatives and doctors didn't want to talk about the mesh scandal in fear of retaliation, or as one doctor said "losing their drinking buddies." Most everyone wanted the subject of mesh to go away and to move on from it so that the real story wouldn't be exposed.

Thank you to all the people who remained anonymous in this story but greatly contributed.

Lastly, to everyone here, who works so hard every day and spends endless hours on the phone talking with people and working for the bigger cause. It is much appreciated.

Jennifer Banmiller

ACKNOWLEDGMENTS

When I began drafting this book in October 2018, the first scene I wrote was of a medical meeting in Chicago, where I met with 15 women who were mesh patients. It was the American Urogynecologic Society's annual "Pelvic Floor Disorders Week" conference—there were lots of big corporate sponsors including makers of vaginal mesh implants.

In interviews, I'd been told how the medical profession was completely dismissive of these women. I'd seen a bit of that cruel, patriarchal behavior in *The Bleeding Edge* documentary by Netflix. Now it was live and in front of me.

Here's what I wrote about the Chicago experience:

> *It is nearly freezing in Chicago, and as the city's nickname says, it's windy.*
>
> *But the women standing outside the Hyatt Regency with their wheelchairs and their anti-mesh protest signs know it's warmer for them out here than inside the hotel. They've been getting icy glares and frosty stares from a number of men through the Hyatt lobby's glass walls.*
>
> *Nearly 1,000 elite—and mostly male—urogynecological physicians are gathered to celebrate the annual "Pelvic Floor Disorders Week" convention, where they'll discuss treatments and operations for ladies with incontinence and sagging pelvises.*

The women have come to Chicago to shout out their anger at the damage done to them by certain lucrative pelvic surgeries such as vaginal mesh implants. The medical association that is running the conference strongly supports vaginal mesh. A number of the association's members on-site are highly paid consultants to the mesh makers; many other physicians at the meeting have become rich from those implants.

The women's banner says, "A mesh injury to one is an injury to all of us." Their T-shirts read "MeshVictimsUnited." One woman's placard says, "Mesh Destroys Lives." And they are chanting "Mesh maims! Mesh kills!"

A doctor in a three-piece suit marches over to the window, looks down the Hyatt's outdoor staircase onto the group of women and pushes a hotel door open.

"What are you doing?" he yells, his words nearly obliterated by the wind. He points down to the "Mesh Destroys Lives" sign and yells again, shaking his head violently at the women. They barely notice him, certainly don't hear him.

They have attracted a small audience that wants to know about this mesh stuff. Conveniently, the women have brought handouts. And little voodoo dolls made of blue plastic mesh that has come out of their pelvises. And photos. Big. Color. Photos. Photos showing plastic mesh stuck in women's abdomens, vaginas, and pelvises.

The doctor—identifiable by the cluster of badges and convention/soiree entry cards hanging around his neck—turns back to the lobby and grabs a hotel employee. He gestures angrily toward the women outside. The hotel worker shrugs his shoulders and the doctor walks off, carrying his official AUGS 2019 conference bag.

The women keep walking with their signs. "So I guess they weren't expecting us," says one of the protestors, Regina. Her friends Katrina and Nancy laugh. A woman named Robin smiles widely at conventioneers walking into the lobby, waving happily. Her head is covered by the only thing she has in her purse to use as a hat in Chicago's cold air: Depend. Those stretchy adult diapers are versatile, and their sophisticated ecru shade works well with Robin's darker coat.

The women—some sitting in wheelable chairs, others with canes—have come from coast to coast to Chicago bound by a terrible curse: vaginal mesh implant injuries. They are all damaged—a missing vagina here, a punctured bladder there, a severed urethra, a permanent limp from injury to the nerves in a leg. They range in age from their 40s to early 60s, but every woman has brought along a pack of diapers.

Almost all the women are strangers to each other. But through one of the many pelvic mesh patient networks—telephone trees and Facebook groups—they have found kinship. Despite difficulties traveling they have come to Chicago to be heard by doctors who have refused to listen to them.

They don't know what they will achieve, but they have at least one agreed-upon goal: a meeting with leaders of the American Urogynecologic Society.

"No one has taken any responsibility for what has happened to us," says Robin. "We need to hear that someone has accountability," she adds, as several of the women nod their heads vigorously.

But they know that outcome is unlikely.

After their meeting that evening with a handful of AUGS folks, including the president and group executive in a room in the hotel's lower floor, the women get on a conference call. They are looking for something positive from the meeting.

"I think that one guy, that doctor, was really surprised when I told him about all the surgeries I've had to repair everything," says Katrina. Yes, but the president didn't seem interested. "He was constantly looking at his watch." Maybe the convention's big kickoff cocktail party in the exhibition hall at the Hyatt was waiting for him to make the opening remarks.

The AUGS people kept saying that their research doesn't show many side effects and that only 1 or 2 percent of the patients have had problems, Katrina says. They said they are going to keep in touch with us, says Nancy.

Are they offering to help pay for mesh repairs? Nope; the women laugh. Are they offering to do mesh removal surgery for free for victims? One of the women just snorts.

"Well, they heard us. They didn't like our signs," Katrina says as the rest of the group chuckles. "I heard that one of the radio stations here did a story on our protest," Robin says.

Indeed. As the women had been entering the meeting room earlier, an AUGS press person was delivering a statement explaining why the medical organization still supports vaginal mesh implants—despite warnings from the FDA.

I mention to the women that leading doctors in the AUGS inner circle complained to me that the media doesn't report on the many women who have had no problems with their mesh. Catcalls come through the phone.

Tomorrow they will go home. And AUGS members will gather for the convention's wrap-up: The Underwater Party at Chicago's giant aquarium. "Celebrating 10 years of karaoke!" says the program, calling the event "AUGSOME."

After Chicago, I could not let go of this book (as my friends will tell you in detail). It was all I could talk about; some people did ask me to stop explaining vaginal mesh during dinner.

So first, I want to thank the women whose tragic stories made this book happen. Regina, Nancy, Katrina, Barbara Lynn, Robin, Marilyn, Dawn, Kath, Caz, Karina, Rose, Billie, Suzanne, "Mary," and many others.

Drs. Dionysios Veronikis, Shlomo Raz, Malcolm Frazer, and Alan Garely gave me a hell of a lot of their valuable time and knowledge. Dr. David Kessler gave me crucial insight.

Dr. Tom Margolis gave me a big push forward. You're right, Tom: men wouldn't put up with this mesh.

Shanin Specter, Kila Baldwin, Katherine Cornell, Ed Blizzard, Cheryl Calderon, and Adam Slater gave me much more than legal explanations.

Jane Akre, you have been a great advocate for all mesh women. Thank you.

The book itself was a team effort. Much thanks to Christina and Benjy. Thank you, Erica, and your anonymous friend—you were invaluable. To my secret sales reps—thanks much.

Bless you, Diana Zuckerman and Jack Mitchell for your information, encouragement, and ideas. David Cay Johnston—you're always on point. To Susan Hergenrather and Ocean Linda, thanks for endless moral support.

I particularly want to thank Dulcy and Richard Hooper for the effort they put into this book as I was writing, and for keeping me focused. And thank you much, Christy, for sending me Rosemary Ramey— Rosemary's extensive experience in medicine and her somewhat-jaundiced insight into the human condition really made this work.

Finally, thank you, Jenn, for this opportunity. I was stunned when I found out how much time and unpaid work you have put into this very personal crusade to help some 200,000 women over the last several years. It's been an adventure and a privilege.

Alicia Mundy
August 2019

IN THEIR OWN WORDS

Insider conversations behind closed doors.

MEDICAL DEVICE MAKERS

"SHOW ME THE MONEY!"
　　—Opening slide in the Johnson & Johnson 2007 PowerPoint
　　　to sales reps on winning domination of the mesh market

"We [sales reps] had, like, scripts designed to highlight the financial benefits of mesh implants. Like, 'See that Lamborghini in the parking lot? That could be YOUR Lamborghini, doctor.'"

"Look, you have to understand these doctors aren't surgeons to begin with; they're obstetricians, so they're not trained in that space. They didn't do that in residency. And they are doing everything blind. Everything by tactile sensation, and by whatever we are telling them," said an ex–sales rep.

"You can implant the mesh in the time it takes to order a Domino's pizza" went the sales reps' script, boasting that this surgery could be performed in 30 minutes or less. "You can do three or four of these implants in a morning and still be on the golf course by noon."

In October 2007, the company [J&J/Ethicon] assessed the "Lessons Learned" from the TVT-Secur experience. Among those lessons cited were "consider not carrying out a first human trial and launching the product at the same time (the learnings from a first human trial should be gathered, digested, and the device/training adjusted accordingly before launch)."

It took them 10 *years* to figure this out?!

FDA AND OTHER MEDICAL AGENCIES

"Since these products are being widely used and successfully marketed with scant published data, there is very little commercial incentive to publish results," the American Urogynecological Society (AUGS) said in its review of its 27th Annual Scientific Meeting.

> Among those lessons cited were "consider not carrying out a first human trial and launching the product at the same time (the learnings from a first human trial should be gathered, digested, and the device/training adjusted accordingly before launch)."

"Without adequate information, the possibility that associated problems will not be identified until a new device has been used on hundreds or possibly thousands of women is significantly increased"
—Conclusion from the above-mentioned AUGS meeting review

"People say the medical device division is 'The Wild West.' Anything goes. Anything can get approved. It's true."
—Former FDA scientist

"The press thinks that the FDA's drug division caves to industry a lot. But it's the medical device office that lets companies walk all over them. For decades."

—Former FDA scientist

"Pelvic mesh? They tested that in rabbits. But not in their pelvises . . . They put a tiny slice of mesh in the rabbit under the skin on its back and its stays there, I don't know, days? If the rabbit doesn't drop dead or turn color, then the plastic is 'biocompatible.' Hey, quit laughing. I'm not kidding."

—Former FDA scientist

Device makers wield more power than drug companies in the FDA and in the Capitol. Several former and current FDA employees have said the device makers don't take no for an answer.

"Given the limited data and frequent changes in marketed products (particularly with regard to the type of mesh material itself, which is most closely associated with several of the postoperative risks, especially mesh erosion), the procedures should be considered *experimental*, and patients should consent to surgery with that understanding."

—Practice Bulletin issued in 2007 by the American College of Obstetricians and Gynecologists (ACOG)

"A growing body of evidence suggests that a small number of patients may have biological responses to certain types of materials in implantable or insertable devices. For example, they develop inflammatory reactions and tissue changes causing pain and other symptoms that may interfere with their quality of life," stated FDA commissioner Scott Gottlieb, MD, and Jeff Shuren, MD, director of the Center for Devices and Radiological Health, in an FDA press release.

Re: 510(k) premarket approval: "That provision, which was meant as an exception, in essence, a little loophole . . . That exception became the rule."

> —Dr. David Kessler, FDA commissioner,
> 1990–97, *The Bleeding Edge*

"So devices can be on the market for years and cause many deaths, many injuries before it becomes public."

> —Madris Tomes, CEO, Device Events, and
> former FDA analyst, *The Bleeding Edge*

DOCTORS

Dr. Matt Barber complained about the many versions of mesh being introduced to market: "We are chasing a moving target."

"I'd never want my wife to have this surgery."

> —Operating room comment from ob-gyn to
> sales rep for J&J pelvic mesh (c. 2006)

"I was putting it [the Tunneller] in and teaching other doctors at the same time," said Dr. Garely. "I put in 12 of them. And I think I had 9 erosions . . . That's when I immediately stopped implanting. I thought, based on the technique of the procedure, I worried I was going to teach someone to kill a patient. I wasn't going to be part of that."

"We should treat implants like medications—the smaller the dose, the fewer side effects. And [we] must have proper clinical trials before you dare to include implants into your practice."

> —Dr. Menahem Neuman

"Unfortunately, through the 510(k) process, we've had some bad products that have been cleared, such as the ObTape . . . and the IVS Tunneller," said Dr. Cheryl Iglesia. "My fear is, in some sense, that I don't want that type of thing to ever hit the market again because that's what leads to the long-term risks."

"What it's like to remove mesh, from the surgeon's perspective, can perhaps be appreciated by this analogy. Extirpation of vaginal mesh is akin to taking a hammer and chisel and trying to remove the rebar from a sidewalk while leaving the cement otherwise intact and not damaging the water mains and power lines below," said Dr. Tom Margolis. "It is difficult, if not impossible, to remove all the mesh and do it safely."

A Canadian study found that 21 percent of those who had to have additional surgeries for TVM revisions had to be treated for depression and almost 3 percent had engaged in "some form of self-harm behaviours, such as attempted suicide, that led to an emergency department visit or admission to a psychiatric hospital."
> —Blayne Welk et al., "Associations of Transvaginal Mesh Complications with the Risk of New-Onset Depression or Self-Harm in Women with a Midurethral Sling," *JAMA*, January 9, 2019

"Most people probably believe that when they get a medical device implanted, be it a pacemaker or a joint, that those medical devices have undergone appropriate testing to demonstrate that they are safe and effective before doctors started using them. But for most moderate and high-risk devices, that is not the case."
> —Dr. Michael Carome, director of Public Citizen's Health Research Group, *The Bleeding Edge*

"It used to be that about 70 percent of biomedical research was funded by the government. In the last 20 to 25 years, that's changed. Now about 70 percent of biomedical research is funded by the industry."
> —Dr. Adriane Fugh-Berman, professor of pharmacology and physiology, Georgetown University, *The Bleeding Edge*

"We can no longer rely on the medical device companies to do what's in the best interest of the patient. And we can no longer rely on the FDA to properly regulate these devices."
—Dr. William Kuo, Stanford Health Care, *The Bleeding Edge*

"I have seen women with their vaginas essentially mutilated. So scarred and disformed as a result of the chronic inflammation and scarring from the mesh as to be left with a nonfunctional vagina or dysfunctional bladder and urethra."
—Dr. Tom Margolis

"When tissue, the vagina, bladder or bowel is damaged enough, no surgeon can fix the tissue past a certain point—and I see that with great regularity, even after mesh was implanted years before."
—Dr. Tom Margolis

LAWYERS

"The core of our objection (to large mass legal fees) is that the cases were settled for way too little and therefore the lawyers are asking for way too much."
—Shanin Specter, plaintiffs' trial attorney, in Law.com, February 2019

"The vast majority of these women were preyed upon by law firms that are marketing and collection firms, and not actual litigation and trial firms," said Adam Slater, trial lawyer who worked with the MDL and shared depositions and discovery from the New Jersey litigation. "Their business model is bad for victims."

"We're going to make millions from this holocaust of pussy."
—Tort attorney from Houston, Texas

"The mesh was defective in many ways. It had way too much plastic. The mesh that's in this box, when you see it, if you unravel it, unravel the mesh that's in this woman's body manufactured by them, that string would reach to the 55th or 56th floor of One Liberty [Philadelphia skyscraper]. I kid you not. 780 feet. *That's 232 feet above William Penn's hat [above City Hall]—all that plastic mesh in her body. And they knew it.*"

—Kline & Specter opening statement in
Prolift case against J&J, 2017

"The women, particularly the most severely injured women who were represented by law firms that never intended to seriously litigate their cases, were the losers in this entire process."

—Adam Slater, plaintiffs' trial attorney, 2019

"Blown SOL's (statute of limitations) are going to be a huge problem."

—Tort attorney from Houston, Texas

THE WOMEN AND THEIR FAMILIES

"My husband began complaining that making love to me was like sleeping with a cheese grater. His penis would be cut when we had intercourse. The pain and embarrassment made me anxious, sick and depressed."

—Mesh survivor in Australia

"My life has been impacted in every way. I am in constant pain, so I cannot do what I used to do, and I must lie down horizontally every hour or so because the pain becomes unbearable. I have experienced bleeding, constant bowel and urination pain, and insomnia every night; I cannot sleep because I am in so much pain. I have always been very active, going to [the] gym, walking, cycling, but everything is very limited now. Every movement hurts. I used to be sexually active prior to this, but now I absolutely cannot. It's just pain, pain, and more pain to merely exist."

—Stella Channing

"I was told by my implanting surgeon that I would be back at the gym within 10 days post-implant procedure and that I would be like a 16-year-old virgin after the implants. To this day, I can't sit upright on a chair for longer than 15 minutes at a time due to the searing pain that travels across my lower abdomen and deep into my pelvis . . . It took a good 14 weeks, not 10 days, post-implant before I was able to get out of bed and walk again. I still, to this very day, experience the same burning pain, even after the removal of both meshes. I describe my pain as being cut open and set alight. It's a deep, burning, searing ache that intensifies with movement."

—Joann

"Add to this my personal experience of trying to teach full-time with a piece of plastic hanging out of an open wound in my vagina for the last three months. I can assure you that it was not just an inconvenience or a trivial or superficial incident."

—Fiona

"The first time we tried to have intercourse it felt like barbed wire inside me. My husband could also feel the mesh. This [came] as a massive shock as my professor had told me I would be like a new woman after childbirth, everything would be tighter. I grieved for my sex life for a long time as my husband and I had only been married 6 months."

—Name withheld

"I was completely bladder incontinent, bowel incontinent; I couldn't have sexual intercourse. I continuously had bladder infections. I developed chronic thrush because of it. I was sick for years. My life revolved around having extra clothes, pads, being close to a toilet and hoping to God that when I had a shower my bowels wouldn't release themselves on me. That was my life."

—Timnat

"By 3 months post-op I was getting pain in my vagina, bleeding and there was mesh eroding out through the side of my Vagina, I noticed a smell that I described as rotting flesh, I went to my GP, who thought

I had a fistula and sent me back to my specialist for review. I saw him and he said it was just a small hiccup, he would 'snip' the small bit of mesh out in his surgery, and he did OMG, it hurt so much and I left, with him telling me to take a couple of Panadol and I would feel OK. This went on for a couple of years, with 4 major surgeries for mesh erosion and multiple trims in his rooms. I was assured this was not very common."

—Name withheld

"I dragged myself to work each day and on weekends I was bedridden. I was unable to do normal things like shopping, cooking, and house-work without debilitating pain and fatigue. My relationship with my family and friends suffered as I could not handle social activities. Not being able to care for my new grandson broke my heart. Surfing was impossible and walking the dogs or doing other light physical exercise was just too painful."

—Name withheld

"How do doctors determine the right outcome?" Kath Sansom asked.

The primary outcome for sling implants is to stop incontinence. "So doctors ask their patients, 'Do you still wet your pants? No—then the implant worked.' They call this success," Kath said.

A number of women who are in the Sling the Mesh advocacy group were injured because the eroding mesh got wound around their coccyx. They have spine issues. They can't walk. They can't sit for hours at a desk. They can't stand up to cook a meal. They're on pain medicines. "Mesh has taken away all the joy from their lives. One woman in 20 on her webpage has said she tried to commit suicide. "There's no escape from pain for them."

"The outcome question should be 'Are you able to resume your normal life?' That's how they should measure success."

INTRODUCTION

What's a vagina worth?

To women, it is a vital part of their essence and the repository that gives life to our species. To men, it is the receptacle that accepts their life-giving sperm and thus creates the greatest mystery of our lives. Birth.

It therefore follows that we should do everything possible, both medically and morally, to protect this most valuable and precious of human interactions from harm. In fact, medical students must take the Hippocratic Oath (or pledge) as an initial step to becoming a doctor, swearing, "First, do no harm."

Unfortunately, as we document in this book, far too many doctors have sworn allegiance to personal profit instead of following the Greek covenant that is one of the oldest binding documents in history, with critical principles that should still be held sacred by doctors.

But doctors were not the original instigators in this conspiracy to turn a serious medical condition into a profitable enterprise. They were, however, the pushers/distributors that medical device makers needed to sell their so-called miracle solutions to women desperate to solve their gynecological problems. These medical cartels, desperate to grow profits through questionable products put into women's bodies, were able to do so thanks to the medical device companies funding the FDA that were unacceptably derelict in their duties when they should have been aggressively protecting women so vulnerable to "quick and safe fixes."

Remember that famous quote from the 1967 film *The Graduate* when a middle-aged man had one word of career advice for Benjamin, the 21-year-old main character? "Plastics . . . there's a great future in plastics." While plastics did become ubiquitous in how products are made, no one then could imagine plastics would one day be inserted into a woman's body as a cure for prolapse, a bulging or falling down body part, such as the rectum or vagina, due to weakened supporting tissues.

The use of plastic vaginal mesh implants expanded into dealing with SUI (stress urinary incontinence) in younger women who developed this bladder problem after having children. Medical device makers began seeing dollar signs and started selling doctors on the idea that the future fix for female incontinence was plastic. Plastic mesh inserts would revolutionize how these doctors treated women for "pelvic floor disorders." Soon, mesh would become the new gold standard for surgery for pelvic organ prolapse and incontinence—conditions that affect a large percentage of women after childbirth and many women over 40.

And the medical device cartel began a concerted sales effort to convince ob-gyns or "baby catchers with a volume business" who could get it in every vagina they inspected, to perform several prolapse repair surgeries a day. Suddenly everyone was talking about mesh and its possibilities, including financial ones. Huge corporations such as Johnson & Johnson were poised to make billions of dollars from pelvic mesh implants. Cha-ching! The medical community came to see the vagina as an ATM.

No wonder the plastic mesh pushers told their sales force and doctors that the risks were minimal—a mere 1 to 2 percent. But that statistic would soon change. In 2017, the United Kingdom, the US, Australia, Scotland, and New Zealand found complication rates of 10 to 15 percent. With three to four million implants globally between 2000 and 2012, that meant several hundred thousand women were having "complications."

Some of those complications were life-changing if not life-threatening: constant incontinence; searing pain that ebbed but didn't end; damage to the bladder, uterus, urethra; nerve and muscle damage caused when the mesh inside the patients began to harden, erode, and "migrate"—the word used to describe pieces of plastic mesh separating inside the pelvis, pushing through vaginal walls, and puncturing organs. When the mesh wrapped itself around the muscles and nerves of their upper thighs, women who had been playing tennis, hiking, swimming, and holding full-time jobs found themselves barely able to walk, relying on wheelchairs and canes. And they couldn't have intercourse after the rogue mesh poked their partners' penises. Once was enough for most men.

And there were deaths—one Missouri woman died about a year after a prolapse mesh implant. She spent most of the intervening time since her 2008 surgery in hospitals, where an infection spread throughout her body. In December 2017, sepsis caused by mesh deterioration claimed the life of this 42-year-old woman from Ontario. But it was not the first death that could be directly linked to vaginal mesh side effects. You will read horrifying stories in this book, including personal accounts of women whose lives have been changed forever.

Patients began searching for surgeons who could take out their mesh, but as one specialist, Dr. Tom Margolis of California, warned US health officials: removing mesh after it had degraded was like trying to remove rebar from concrete.

It's the template for every medical scandal: the FDA was derelict in its duties, industry lobbying groups held the FDA hostage, and the companies knew much more than they revealed when initially marketing their meshes. Whether the issue was a pharmaceutical product, medical device, or hospital failure, the process was the same—people

> It's the template for every medical scandal: the FDA was derelict in its duties, industry lobbying groups held the FDA hostage, and the companies knew much more than they revealed when initially marketing their meshes.

knew the problem and they reported it, but it was dismissed in favor of meeting company growth goals and keeping revenue promises to investors.

It took lawsuits, as usual, to uncover the truth. The truth was ugly. Internal memos within the companies showed detailed knowledge not only of potential risks but records of repeated failures using the new products. When the legal fights were over, companies continued earning blockbuster profits. And regulatory officials in the US and elsewhere who had monitored the medical crisis—in this case, vaginal mesh—ended up with high-paying jobs in the very companies they had been "regulating."

And the lawyers didn't start the fire, but they saw dollar signs in signing up helpless victims. Along the way, some law firms anxious to settle short-changed victims by pressuring them to "just take the money" so they could collect their cut and, for some, very lucrative leadership fees.

Sadly, as you will read, there is plenty of blame to go around. Our fervent hope is that this book will in some small measure be the voice crying out for the thousands of women victimized by this medical scandal that never should have happened.

CHAPTER 1

CAPITALISM GONE WILD

"SHOW ME THE MONEY!"

—Opening slide in the Johnson & Johnson 2007 PowerPoint to
sales reps on winning domination of the mesh market

This is a story about greed.

It's about a massive medical industry campaign to make a huge profit from patients, aided and abetted by doctors across the country.

It's about a two-decades-long cover-up of serious injuries, including deaths, caused by products that should never have been widely prescribed for humans.

It's about the willingness to ignore evidence about damages from these products to patients—and their families—in order to meet corporate marketing algorithms that will cause revenues to skyrocket.

It's about the crisis caused by these products to the American health-care system and the hundreds of thousands of patients who need major medical treatment to recover.

No, it's not about the opioid or JUUL epidemic.

It's about pelvic mesh and its victims. But the addicts in this scandal are the makers and the sellers—the corporations and the doctors— so desperate for a fix of cash that they will sell their product anyplace, anytime, and to anyone they can.

Medical disasters happen. People make mistakes.

But that wasn't the case with vaginal mesh.

Vaginal mesh is a classic medical product scandal driven by a group of health-care corporations and their particularly profitable "Women's Health" divisions. There are unexpected twists in the plot, including the appearance of many doctors and lawyers in surprising roles as villains. The size and scalability are also unique.

> Women's reproductive organs are the most lucrative medical device moneymakers that exist.

The one non-surprise is that the corporations, such as Johnson & Johnson and Boston Scientific, knew in advance that their medical products—in this case, vaginal mesh implants—could cause serious permanent damage to women, and at higher numbers than their published "risk" rates. In true medical product scandals, companies always know.

Women's reproductive organs are the most lucrative medical device moneymakers that exist. Issues such as bladder leakage, bad sex from vaginal dryness, birth control complications, and urinary tract infections can cause fear that your partner will leave you or have an affair because having sex is different. Wrinkles, weight gain, vaginal leakage or prolapse, and any problems with the pelvis can compound common insecurities we have about getting older.

Women were played by these companies and their sales representatives—which included doctors and their elite professional medical organizations. Some two million women in America (about four million women globally) had vaginal mesh implants either for incontinence or prolapse (or both). And if data from countries such as the United Kingdom and Australia are correct, about 10 percent of these patients have already developed or will (perhaps even years from now) develop "complications" from those implant surgeries.

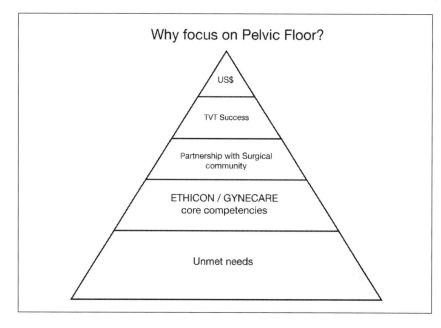

Why focus on Pelvic Floor?

US$

TVT Success

Partnership with Surgical community

ETHICON / GYNECARE core competencies

Unmet needs

Not all the patients will have serious, debilitating, or permanent injuries. But there will be many more cases of severe damage than companies estimated when they were pushing their expensive marketing campaigns. Many women with those severe injuries have needed multiple operations—sometimes up to 10 surgeries—to correct damage done by mesh to other organs or to leg muscles, and many of them will never be able to have sex again.

The medical bills are hefty. Someone will have to pay them. It shouldn't be the women.

The 1970s brought women's liberation and revolution. Women were holding jobs outside the home. They were also looking younger longer and staying active longer. The definition of aging had changed.

Thanks to new facial care products and the exponential growth and falling costs of cosmetic surgery, women could tell their faces and bosoms that "age is just a number."

But try telling that to your vagina. Or your bladder. Tell your 50-year-old pelvis it's still 30.

Some women tried, but their bodies weren't listening. There were side effects to staying younger longer, to having a career and visibility in the community or the corporate world.

For instance: you move, you lose. Same for laughing or coughing. With SUI there's leakage, peeing your pants, a feeling that something's slowly dropping out of you. Times had changed, but the female anatomy hadn't.

The only options for serious incontinence or prolapse were versions of major surgery called the Burch procedure. It took more than an hour, sometimes two; involved an abdominal incision; the insertion of a small support hammock made of "native" tissue—perhaps one of your leg tendons, perhaps one from an animal or human cadaver; sutures to hold up the organs that were drooping or pressing upon the bladder; and several days' recovery in the hospital.

Needless to say, women weren't standing in lines for these operations and doctors weren't becoming rich from them.

Then, in the 1990s, doctors began toying with the idea of using a synthetic material for the support, or hammock, and performing a less invasive surgical procedure to lift the pelvic organs.

There are some wild tales and horror stories about the advent of these innovations. Basically, the guys in white coats said, "Well, hernia mesh is a big success; let's put it in the pelvis. And we can take a shortcut. We'll go in through the vagina!"

There's a lot to say about this. For now, it's important to know just one big thing to understand why pelvic mesh implants caused so much damage.

The scientists and doctors and companies didn't test the mesh in vaginas first.

That's right. They just started making and selling it. Women were the guinea pigs.

Like all medical product scandals, the mesh disaster could have been controlled. After the first incontinence sling was recalled by the company in 1997 (a humiliation for Boston Scientific), the five companies rushing to own a piece of the nascent vaginal mesh market should have hit "pause" in their labs while they figured things out.

The US Food and Drug Administration should have also cautioned companies waiting for FDA approval to sell their new meshes. There should have been some warning to the public.

The doctors "consulting" with the medical device companies and the national medical organizations helping those companies market mesh to meet the "unmet needs" of women should have called a "time-out" while they reviewed the problems with vaginal mesh.

But patients were kept in the dark. The major corporations, which are dependent on their investors, refused to admit that they had known about the dangers from their mesh implants. Nor did they admit that the risks of damage, even permanent injury, were much higher than they had told doctors whom they recruited to their sales scheme.

There was a white wall—the medical wall of silence. The corporations could pull this off because too many American doctors—urologists and women's go-to physicians, their ob-gyns—were complicit in this. So were their medical professional organizations that are

> The mesh makers knew that they would be protected by our prurience, our embarrassment about making news about vaginas, particularly aging vaginas and incontinence.

heavily funded by medical companies. And though a federal regulator's job is to protect consumers from dangerous health-care products, the FDA publicly maintained the corporate message: pelvic mesh is effective and safe, and its complications are rare. The agency did this for a full decade before the first official (and wimpy) warning.

Guess who else added to the silence that kept women from learning about mesh problems? The media.

Can you recall a medical product disaster affecting 100,000 or more women that would not lead to 24/7 news coverage for a week, congressional hearings, and at least one criminal investigation?

When it comes to public discussion, "vagina" remains taboo. "Pelvic mesh" sounds more palatable, but still something that makes people squirm and change the subject.

The mesh makers knew that they would be protected by our prurience, our embarrassment about making news about vaginas, particularly aging vaginas and incontinence.

Asked why newspapers don't focus on more stories about corruption involving large drug and medical device companies, and about mesh in particular, a reporter for a national daily said, "Because we know they are corrupt, so it's not news!"

That's true. Those companies also spend billions of dollars on advertising, which locks them up with the media companies—TV, newspapers, magazines. Few TV networks or cable outlets are willing to risk losing those ad dollars from medical companies unless the issue involves cancer or children. One of the only media companies to take on mesh was Netflix, whose 2018 documentary *The Bleeding Edge*, included some graphic details about the surgeries, the injuries, and the married couples who couldn't have sex anymore.

The TV news show *60 Minutes* did a segment involving counterfeit plastic mesh material imported from China by Boston Scientific, but the coverage focused on the business scheme and quickly got away from anatomical references.

There's another reason mesh hasn't had a lot of news attention. It's a complicated story: There isn't just one health-care corporation involved but a half dozen. And there are at least 12 different products. Still, it takes just one to ruin a woman's life.

As for congressional hearings—anyone who's worked around politicians, particularly the aging white males on Capitol Hill and in statehouses, knows how little they would welcome the chance to say "vaginas" in front of C-Span and America.

This is a real problem, because the mesh disaster is not over yet. For some, it hasn't even begun, but it will. Many women who had mesh implants are still symptom-free: no pain, no chronic UTI, no tissue-necrotizing infections in their pelvis, no loss of the ability to walk, no pieces of hardened plastic sticking through their vaginal walls and injuring their partners during intercourse.

These women may not develop serious problems until 10 years after their implants. What will they do if they suddenly develop the symptoms listed above and aren't aware that mesh can erode and cause all those problems?

What if that happened to you, years after "minor" outpatient mesh surgery? What would you do?

Would you know the mesh was the cause of your medical problem? Would your doctor? Would you know how to find your old medical records? Would you know how to find the right care? Would your insurance or Medicare be willing to cover major medical treatment for side effects from an old elective procedure?

For thousands of American women, that answer has been no.

We know that because we've spoken to tens of thousands of women over the last six years concerning their mesh implants. They've been bounced from doctor to doctor, trying to get answers. Many women have been told their problems were in their heads, though they were all quite sure the pain was much lower than that, in their vaginas.

The medical device industry played women, played their insecurities about their appearance and their acceptability to men. Mesh can't cure weight or wrinkles, but it was marketed and advertised in a way to cure just about everything else—a real fountain of youth.

GREED IS GOOD

What made mesh especially appealing for the medical device industry was the scalability of it. There are millions of women to go after; there are thousands of doctors who had hundreds of patients that they could recruit for mesh implants; and there were no limitations for vaginal mesh use anywhere in the world. Cha-ching: $$$!

The future of female incontinence was plastic. Plastic mesh inserts were already revolutionizing how doctors treated women for incontinence. Soon mesh would become the new gold standard for prolapse surgery—problems with a large demographic, roughly 25 percent of women over 40.

In Paris at a 2004 conference of influential urogynecologists, plastics—specifically plastic mesh—was the hot topic. Mesh makers sponsoring the tony affair were strategizing ways to expand the vaginal mesh market in America and Europe with the International Urogynecological Association and the International Continence Society.

A feast for the doctors was held at a place synonymous with greed: Versailles, the historic palace of festivals and peace treaties. One of the organizations' newsletters chronicled the high points: "It was a very successful meeting aided by superb conference facilities at the Palais des Congrès, and the fact that Paris is Paris. The Gala Dinner was held at the Palais de Versailles, and commenced with drinks and nibbles on the steps overlooking the sweep of gardens and fountains while the sun set along the avenue of fountains. Behind were the buildings of the palace. The dinner itself was held in the historic Orangerie." The evening ended with fireworks that exploded over the palace gardens where Marie Antoinette once frolicked at a costume ball dressed as a shepherdess.

During the conference, one doctor from France announced that the world of urogynecology was about to be upended by a new wave of plastic surgical devices for pelvic organ prolapse. The speaker, Dr. Michel Cosson, told his audience that this was the time to join the movement. Urogynecologists would be able to perform several pro-lapse mesh implants a day. Dr. Cosson, a well-paid consultant for Johnson & Johnson's Ethicon, had to pull himself away from all the doctors at the session trying to talk with him.

"Everyone was talking about mesh," said a guest in an interview for this book. No one at the conference talked about the dangers, said the guest. The risks, if anyone asked the companies or their consultants, were minimal—only 1 to 2 percent.

Meanwhile, these women were searching for surgeons who could remove their mesh. But as one specialist in such surgery, Dr. Tom Margolis of California, had warned the Food and Drug Administration: removing mesh after it had degraded was like trying to remove rebar from concrete.

THE MEDICAL DEVICE MAKERS'
MEGALOMANIA

That's the medical device industry and its pushers among physicians. It's all about the money.

It's almost impossible for average patients, even for policy makers, to change that. That is because medical device makers have the most power in this country in terms of what they can do with their reckless disregard for human life. They can insulate themselves from legal issues, pay off the lobbyists they own, and even manipulate the FDA—which is funded by medical device and drug companies. It's not a stretch to say that they operate like real-life drug cartels, run from big executive offices in New Jersey, Minnesota, and Massachusetts, in plain sight with logos we all love and buy from because we trust them.

"People think pharma's got power," said Jim Spencer, journalist at the Minneapolis *Star Tribune*, in *The Bleeding Edge*. "No, no, no, no. The device industry has much more power than pharma."

Even in litigations similar to that for mesh, millionaire lawyers who chase billionaire medical device makers are always on an uneven playing field. Medical device makers stall, refusing to turn over documents until they are forced by court. In some cases, documents disappear, as many did at Ethicon. Mesh makers have been untouchable and protected by everyone from legislators to the media, from doctors to our executive branch.

This story is about the women who, on a daily basis, have to live with the eroded, painful device. Many will never fully recover due to the nerve damage from multiple surgeries or the particles of plastic that are so imbedded in their tissues that they cannot be removed. An alarming number of women globally have also developed symptoms of autoimmune diseases such as lupus, which the companies insist aren't related to mesh.

Thousands of women affected by mesh have stories such as these. They trusted their doctors, with whom they had a history, because physicians are the ones with the medical degrees. They were told that this simple procedure would easily cure their embarrassing female issues. After the surgery, these women wanted—no, needed—to get help to solve these unbearable issues with pain, fatigue, depression, and more, but they had no idea what the cause of their symptoms was. They were either too scared, too tired, or too embarrassed to fight on their own behalf.

Blatant sexism has played a role in the way that the medical industry as a whole has responded to victims, brushing off their complaints of pain as female hysteria and weakness. As one mesh survivor named Robin poignantly shared, "I question who I am, at the loss of my vagina. So emotionally traumatized by this, yet shown no empathy by medical personnel where I live . . . Instead, after life-altering surgery, I have been treated as a spectacle of curiosity, with no answers to future treatment."

Furthermore, many, if not most, of the doctors who did implants were never properly trained. Nonetheless, they made their practices into drive-thru surgery centers. Mesh implants were supposedly quick and easy procedures, and they promised an endless supply of profits, much more than the standard duties associated with traditional ob-gyn work.

> Would you want a surgical procedure performed by a doctor who learned what to do from a YouTube video?

What should have been left to experienced surgeons was put into the hands of doctors who had no idea what they were doing and no way of fixing the problems they created.

Would you want a surgical procedure performed by a doctor who learned what to do from a YouTube video? What if you knew that your doctor learned this "skill" at a weekend conference where he was the 50th doctor in line to put the device in the same cadaver?

It's no wonder that women were irreparably injured when the doctors were slicing their flesh and tugging strips of plastic back and forth in the pelvis. It would be more shocking if these training methods worked.

The FDA failed to require proper testing before putting mesh in the vagina. They were beyond derelict in their duties, and after the first transvaginal mesh incontinence product ProteGen was recalled, federal regulators allowed subsequent versions to be fast-tracked to market, despite the product's significant potential to damage countless patients.

And the drug lords—medical device makers—played real-life Monopoly with an industry that strives to move ahead of competitors, buys up the most doctors through weekend getaways and luxury cars, and makes obscenely high profits, using their "Get Out of Jail Free" card. Not one CEO has been put behind bars, or even investigated, for the destruction of so many lives.

ROBIN'S STORY

What do you call a journey that involves five hospitals, 75 doctors, takes 13 years, 12,000 miles in trips, and includes a neo-vagina?

You call it Robin's life since vaginal mesh. Millions of women have mesh, and Robin is one of the tens of thousands who have been irreparably harmed by it. These women are why this story of greed, a broken system, and sexism needs to be told. To fully understand this tale, it's first critical to know the intense emotional, physical, and mental agony that these survivors have been battling on a daily basis for years.

"Hey, when I go to a medical center, I'm very popular. Every doctor wants to meet me. They don't want to meet me, really; they just want to get a look at my neo-vagina. But I like to think of it as a way to make new friends," says Robin.

Robin has a knack for sarcasm. In fact, sarcasm is her oxygen. "If I couldn't make jokes about some of this, I'd be dead," she explains.

One of the mesh women called Robin "the canary in the coal mine." She meant that Robin is the entity whose problems—and whose outcome—will indicate just how bad things are for the rest of the women in the same situation. She's right.

Robin's story is a cautionary tale for women with very serious injuries from vaginal mesh and whose damages can never be fully repaired because the situation is not going to get any better.

Your lawyers are going to get tired. Your doctors are going to move on, mentally if not physically. Your only option may be a treatment that doesn't have a Medicare billing code: misery management.

Meandering Mesh

Once upon a time, Robin had a life. She attended four different colleges due to her husband's US Air Force military career. On Guam, because the on-base elementary schools were disappointing, she homeschooled her children. Then she was asked by other American parents abroad to set up homeschooling support groups.

When she and her family moved back to the US, Robin graduated from homeschooling to teaching in schools. "I enjoyed it, I connected with the kids, and I was good," Robin says.

Her own four children grew up, and Robin branched out. She got her real estate license and cosmetology license. She also took up aerobics and became an instructor. And she was still in her 40s.

But you've already guessed what comes next.

In 2006, Robin had surgery at a US military hospital for incontinence. Like a number of women, she says she was not told she would have permanent plastic implants attached inside her pelvic area. The doctor and Robin discussed a bladder suspension, using sutures, and she thought that's what was being done at Fort Carson.

Within months of that first surgery, after a Monarc sling made by American Medical Systems was implanted, her physical situation deteriorated. But she wasn't told about the sling.

After the surgery she had immediate problems. For instance, Robin said, "I was peeing like a man—the urine spray between the seat and the bowl. It went everywhere." Her doctor told her, "Don't worry, Mrs. B. It will all loosen up."

"I had no clue that it was a mesh sling," she said. Nor did she know it had already begun eroding. Or that her urethra, which controls the direction of the urine stream, was damaged.

During 2007 and 2008, Robin was having constant burning vaginosis and discomfort in her groin. Other gynecologists examining her vaginally "felt" something, but didn't discuss what this was. (Hint: mesh erosion.)

The burning vaginosis worsened and infected her husband Carl. The result? Testing of both Robin and Carl for STDs, HIV, hepatitis C—and the bonus question was when the doctors asked her husband about his sexual habits.

Carl hadn't hit the high point yet. A few months later, his penis was grazed and abraded during intercourse by Robin's meandering mesh—the mesh she still did not know she had. She couldn't eat, and her most comfortable position was fetal.

Meanwhile, her white cell count began skyrocketing. She was sent to Rocky Mountain Oncology Center, getting blood tests every two weeks. There was a bone marrow biopsy, one of the more painful medical tests. One doctor told her she had leukemia. But she didn't.

"I couldn't eat the way I used to. I asked my doctors if they thought I had developed celiac disease."

"Oh no," they said.

"But I put myself on a celiac diet"—meaning no gluten, among other restrictions. Her white cell count dropped out of "leukemia" range. And she didn't get sick after eating anymore.

"But when I was given a medicine—a pill that we learned contained gluten binder—I suddenly broke out into a burning rash," Robin says.

Like other mesh victims, Robin developed urinary tract infections. She had so many UTIs that she needed almost a regular supply of antibiotics. "But now I needed antibiotics that come in liquid form so that it's not in a tablet with gluten binders." In 2010, one of her blood tests showed she was positive for celiac, but Robin was too tired to say, "I told you so."

Her lower abdomen and groin were sore. The former aerobic instructor couldn't lift her newborn granddaughter. "I couldn't lift anything over 10 pounds without feeling like my gut was pulling out."

Her increasingly unusual symptoms had her bouncing from doctor to doctor. She began developing resistance to the antibiotics she was using, which was problematic because she had constant UTIs and vaginitis.

Meanwhile, the main problem that had started Robin's saga—incontinence—was out of control. "I had such incontinence that if I stood up, urine ran out of me," Robin says. "I wore adult diapers almost constantly."

"I still didn't know I had a Monarc implant in me. I went to gynecologists and complained about the constant and severe pain during sex, and they said they felt something in my vagina pushing out. They would give me estrogen cream, which soothes the skin there and thickens the tissue," she explains. But that didn't work for long.

A new gynecologist she visited in Colorado Springs suggested surgery using mesh. "I'd started hearing about mesh problems and told him I didn't want it."

But the doctor said it was the "new" improved mesh and the best way to treat incontinence. That surgery, which involved an Ethicon TVT sling, took place in March 2012. After the surgery, she was in severe pain, with a hematoma in her bladder, and she couldn't sit up. The doctor told her, "You're a bleeder." It took eight weeks to recover. "I was in bed from March to May that year," Robin sighed.

Interestingly, that gynecologist who implanted the TVT sling either did not notice there was already an incontinence sling inside Robin—the AMS Monarc—or he just didn't think to mention it.

Robin shopped for other gynecologists. The UTIs and vaginitis worsened. Robin and Carl went to one doctor together because between Robin's pain, the scratches to his penis, and the eternal infections, having sex—for Mr. and Mrs. B.—was becoming a risky enterprise.

One urologist told Robin that she should never have had the TVT sling put in. He recommended urethra blockers. She declined.

A female gynecologist told Robin she could "fix" her by putting in many stitches. But the pain was worsening and the UTI-vaginitis combo was raging. Robin and Carl visited the doctor together to ask what the heck was happening. "The doctor yelled at me and my husband. She said, "I DID NOT DO THIS TO YOU!" The doctor seemed scared that Mr. and Mrs. B. might be trying to pin liability for something on her. "My husband said to her, 'Hey, we haven't mentioned lawyers! We just want to know what's wrong.'"

The next doctor told Robin, "You've got a lot of damage." But, he said, he couldn't remove the sling in her because it would cause her more damage.

Robin started 2013 with more incontinence and went back to her primary care doctor. "She wasn't listening to me. I told her I was having more stabbing pain. It felt like a knife was in my vagina. I couldn't get out of bed."

Robin tried explaining it in more detail to her doctor. "If you took a kettlebell and clipped it to a man's scrotum, it would feel like that, with the weight pulling down my vagina. It was horrible."

Robin told her primary care doctor that she wanted to see another gynecologist. But with Tricare insurance, Robin needed another referral which meant waiting because the doctor had to provide a legitimate reason for the referral. "It wasn't enough that I described what it felt like."

"Finally, I took a picture of my rear end," said Robin. "By this time I could see that in my vaginal area, something was slipping out. I showed the photo to my primary care doctor, and she got me a referral to a urogynecologist."

The urogynecologist, who was at a large Colorado hospital, said Robin would need to have her pelvis and some other organs pulled up into place.

"He told me that the picture I took was my small intestine slipping out of me. I went into the restroom in his office and threw up. I didn't know this could happen," Robin said.

Revenge Fantasies

Robin had had it.

"I'd been getting gaslighted," she said. That's a reference to the famous 1944 movie *Gaslight*, where the nasty husband played by Charles Boyer tries to drive his innocent wife, played by Ingrid Bergman, crazy to get her money. He kept telling the Ingrid character that she was seeing things that weren't there—when they really were. In one frightening scene, Ingrid tells Charles, "You think I'm insane, don't you!?"

"That's what had been happening to me, and to a lot of other women," Robin said.

They told her: "Mrs. B., this isn't physical. Nothing's moving around inside you. There's nothing hanging out of you."

Or "Mrs. B., you need to see a counselor. This is all in your head."

"One time I was so angry with a doctor saying that, that I was tempted to take off my diaper and pee on his shiny office floor. But that really would have seemed psychotic, so I didn't. But I wanted to. A revenge fantasy." Robin laughed.

In 2015, Robin had both urine and fecal incontinence. Another doctor in a Denver hospital suggested a sacrocolpopexy procedure. "She examined me lying down, and said, 'Oh my gosh!'"

The doctor asked Robin to stand up so she could better examine what was going on with Robin's pelvic and rectal areas to determine the extent of Robin's prolapse. "She said, 'Oh my God, it's coming out of you!'"

"She took me and my husband into a room to talk with us. She also wanted to put in mesh, and she was pushing the daVinci robot method to implant it. I said no."

Robin was now in so much pain, she quit her job in computer data input on the military base. She turned to the Internet. She found an online group of US mesh patients—victims—and talked with one. The lady recommended Robin contact Dr. Shlomo Raz at UCLA. Robin made an appointment with him.

Before going to Dr. Raz, Robin contacted a law firm in Houston that advertised they handle mesh cases. They told her to get all her medical records collected. "And that's how I found out that I had TWO meshes in me. That's when I learned the Monarc sling had been implanted with the first doctor in 2006, when I thought he was doing a 'suspension' surgery."

Robin flew to Los Angeles in June 2015. "Dr. Raz examined me and said, 'Not only do you have serious pelvic prolapse, but your rectum and your bladder are coming out of you.'"

The medical term is "inversion."

"The organs in my pelvic area and my groin were starting to hang out of me," Robin said.

Dr. Raz reviewed Robin's rather extensive medical history dating back to 2006. "He told me that he thought a lot of my autoimmune issues—like the rashes and the allergies I have—are linked to the mesh. Probably getting the mesh out would help that subside. He also said he believed mesh is pre-contaminated. Before it goes in, there's bacteria already."

Over the course of the next 23 months, Dr. Raz performed five surgeries on Robin.

To prepare, Raz removed ligaments from Robin's thighs to create grafts of "native tissue" for the operations. "Swimsuit competitions are out now," she said, showing the three 10-inch scars on her thighs. One ligament piece was used to help repair her urethra. "He cut it in half, made it like a straw and used extra ligaments to support it," she explained. Dr. Raz also had to make a graft to support her sphincter muscle, which was damaged.

After the first surgery in December 2015, Raz told Robin that the mesh erosion and damage to tissue and organs he found inside her was far worse than he thought when he initially examined her a few months earlier.

"You are among the top 10 worst mesh cases I've ever seen," he told me.

With the surgery, Robin recalled, "I went into septic shock—Dr. Raz said there was lots of bacteria on the mesh. I needed five transfusions. While I was in the recovery room, my husband was watching and said I was turning blue. I was in the ICU seven days. There was a giant hematoma in my pelvic area and groin."

Dr. Raz told Robin he could not proceed with the next steps, including pelvic reconstruction, because of all the trauma to her body from the initial operation. She needed more recovery time.

With much of her mesh now removed, Robin became completely incontinent. "I couldn't feel when I was peeing." Once, when the pee just came out of her in a public place, she told Carl, "I'm just marking my territory."

The second surgery with Dr. Raz took place five months later. "That's when he told me he had found both the Monarc and the TVT in me. Dr. Raz said he had never seen anything like this before."

"The mesh had gone through my urethra and was starting to barrel through my bladder. My vaginal tissue was shredding in places, and my rectum was prolapsing."

From 2015 through 2017, Robin and her husband made 11 trips to UCLA from Denver. "It was all out-of-pocket expenses. We had to stay somewhere. And we paid for a lot of the medical things insurance didn't cover. My husband had to take unpaid leave. I think between his not working, my not working, and all the things we paid for out of pocket, it's probably cost us $150,000."

At one point Robin was in bed for over eight weeks.

"Little" problems became disasters. "Dr. Raz had given me an antibiotic prescription for home, and after I took it, I got a big rash. It was Bactrim. I don't know if it had gluten in it. I found out that for some reason, they couldn't find the reference to celiac disease in my Tricare records. My primary care doctor in Colorado prescribed something else, and I had another reaction. But my primary care doctor would not provide me with a 'brand-name-only' prescription," she said.

"It took me calling my congressman (Republican Doug Lamborn). One of the lawyers in his office, Dave Anderson, contacted Tricare and explained I had a medical necessity to have a brand name, and they agreed. Dr. Raz sent a new prescription. And that's how I got the right antibiotic."

It's Complicated

In May 2016, Robin was set for her second operation with Raz. The incident over the brand-name antibiotic prescription came back to bite Robin. She said that a couple of weeks before the surgery in Los Angeles, "My primary care doctor in Colorado sends a letter saying she doesn't want to treat me anymore."

Robin had to find another primary care physician before she left for UCLA. On May 2, 2016, Dr. Raz did "everything"— rectocele, cystocele, the full vaginal vault. Robin had physical reactions to the pain medication and was in the hospital for seven days. "Dr. Raz said, 'You are so complicated.'"

Two weeks later, the bladder was still prolapsing, even after Dr. Raz used Robin's native tissue—from her leg ligaments—to rebuild something to support the bladder. "It was very, very painful," says Robin. "And then the nurse came in to tell me my roommate complained that I kept her awake because I was crying in my sleep!"

In December 2016, Dr. Raz created a spiral sling, like a ribbon, to support Robin's prolapsed bladder. "But I was becoming allergic to the pain medicine, codeine and Tylenol. My liver was, like, shutting down—my ALT score (liver test) went up to 632 and the GI surgeon wanted to biopsy my liver. I refused a biopsy. I said, 'Nope, I think it's probably the Tylenol. I took myself off it, and the liver reading relaxed. But I have problems taking opiates, too."

Here's how Robin tested herself for Tylenol interaction. During this time she had a terrible flu and had been taking Mucinex as well as the pain medicine. She switched to Mucinex without the Tylenol. "My liver tests changed. That was it."

After that surgery, Dr. Raz said Robin had vaginal shortening and had suffered so much erosion that she'd essentially lost her vagina. "Carl and I couldn't have intercourse. I'm very lucky my husband didn't walk out the door like some other husbands have done."

Dr. Raz told her she was too young not to ever have sex again.

"I wanted a neovagina. I researched it online. I had just met a new urologist, but he told me I was 'too complicated' for that operation. I called another doctor in October 2017 and explained what I wanted. The doctor, a female, mentioned she was pregnant. But when I said I wanted to find someone who could make a neovagina for me, she said, 'Mrs. B., why would you want to do this?' I said, 'I would like my life back.' There was silence on the phone. Then she said, 'OK,'" and told Robin to go back to Dr. Raz and see a sex therapist.

"Dr. Raz did the neovagina, repaired my herniated bladder, found even more frayed mesh in me. I still have some. I was in the hospital for two weeks, and had an autoimmune reaction. Dr. Raz said I was the most complicated patient he'd ever had. He chalked it up to the biofilm on the mesh that was full of bacteria."

There are Costco-size containers of Depend diapers in her house in Colorado Springs.

Since 2017 Robin has been dealing with various primary care doctors and assorted surgeons and urologists. She's also contacted doctors who work with the transgender community and therefore have experience with "neovaginas," and who might be able to fix slipping neovaginas. But the transgender community apparently doesn't have this particular kind of neovagina. It's rarely done, Robin explained. She didn't have stomach muscles left that could be used to make it because the mesh had damaged those muscles, so Dr. Raz had to improvise.

"Do you believe this!? I go to the transgender-community experts on building vaginas. And transgender-sex-change surgeons tell me that *my case* is unusual."

She's also got doctors who think antibiotics are not the way to treat urinary tract infections. Also, hospitals that demand referral slips to make appointments with their specialists, even when Tricare Select tells them the patient has the Select plan and does not need a referral.

"It's institutional euthanasia," says Robin. "They want to see how much I can spin around before I drop. And I'm not alone.

"My outlook is simple. Every day's a different shade of gray. I am always going to have pain and incontinence. It's not a pretty story," Robin adds.

"I've thought about calling the suicide hotline," she says, pausing. "But I don't want to make those people get depressed . . ."

CHAPTER 2

HOW THE DEAL WENT DOWN

"Devices can be on the market for years and cause
many deaths, many injuries before it becomes public."

—Madris Tomes, CEO, Device Events, and former FDA analyst, *The Bleeding Edge*

"We can no longer rely on the medical device
companies to do what's in the best interest of
the patient. And we can no longer rely on the
FDA to properly regulate these devices."

—Dr. William Kuo, Stanford Health Care, *The Bleeding Edge*

Like all historical events and great scandals in history, transvaginal mesh took decades of deceit and involved countless players to snowball into this epic crime against women. To explain all this, it's necessary to get a quick history of how a certain kind of plastic ended up in millions of women's vaginas.

POLYPROPYLENE: IF IT'S GOOD ENOUGH FOR FISHING LINE, IT'S GOOD ENOUGH FOR SURGERY

To understand why vaginal mesh was going to damage the body, you need a clear picture of polypropylene, the plastic threads that are woven together to create mesh products. Polypropylene was first polymerized (a chemical reaction that combines two or more molecules to form larger molecules that contain repeating structures) in 1951 by a pair of scientists at Phillips Petroleum. After World War II, the demand for oil products was diminishing. So the company had to search for other methods to turn their vast quantities of natural gas into a new product to make money.

While trying to figure out how to convert ethylene and propylene—hydrocarbons produced when refining natural gas—into components for gasoline, they found a way to make a solid and unique resin. They called it high-density polyethylene (HDPE); it was a far stiffer, harder, and more heat-resistant material than anything available on the market at that time. This is basically the conception of the modern world of plastics as we know it.

Phillips marketed this new material under the name Marlex Polyethylene. Guess what child's toy brought this strong plastic to popularity? The Hula-Hoop! The proceeds from this highly popular product allowed Phillips to create different grades of Marlex that could be manufactured for a variety of uses. Soon its ability to be sterilized at high temperatures made it a preferred choice for baby bottles and other food containers.

Interestingly enough, three separate research teams had created polypropylene in different labs within a short time of each other. Between 1951 and 1953, three patent applications on the discovery of polypropylene were filed: one by a team from Phillips; one from Standard Oil; and one from Karl Ziegler of the Max Planck Institute. Starting in 1958, a nearly three-decade battle ensued involving the US Patent and Trademark Office. Many scientists were in favor of Professor Ziegler and Italian scientist Giulio Natta to win the patent because their groundbreaking work and publications on polymers led to them receiving the Nobel Prize. But in 1983, the patent went to the scientists from Phillips.

POLYPROPYLENE AS SURGICAL MESH

Polypropylene was soon found to have many benefits: it doesn't absorb water; it can be spun into a threadlike material and dyed any color; it's lightweight and flexible; and it won't shatter.

Currently, polypropylene can be found everywhere including in toys, food containers, fabrics, upholstery, tech devices, fishing line, and more. It was worth $81.6 billion in 2014 and is projected to reach $133.3 billion by 2023.

With such an innovative product, it seemed like a brilliant idea to use it for medical procedures, so soon it was tried in hernia repair surgery. A hernia occurs when an organ or fatty tissue squeezes through a weak spot in the surrounding muscle. In the 1900s, various forms of woven soft metal grafts were used to reinforce this tear to prevent the tissue from pushing out. Repair can be executed in two ways: sewing the tissue of the abdominal wall using sutures, or by placing mesh to cover the hernia defect and reinforcing surrounding tissue with fibrin glue, staples, or sutures.

In the mid-1950s, medical researchers studied the use of "modern" materials such as nylon, Orlon, Dacron, and Teflon. But these caused negative reactions in the body.

New articles touting Marlex encouraged scientists to work with that plastic, and a woven mesh was developed. In 1958, a doctor named Francis Usher published his surgical technique using a polypropylene mesh. Just 30 years later, success with Marlex mesh was reported in a study involving 6,321 hernia patients. Surgical mesh seemed to be the answer that so many medical researchers had been looking for—so where else could it be used?

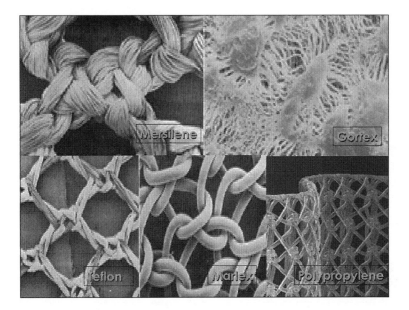

ULF ULMSTEN: THE FATHER OF PELVIC MESH

One man had an idea about where to next put Marlex, and he went to work on it in the early 1990s. By the time the pelvic mesh craze was sweeping America, 1998–2005, few people were cheering louder for this new device than Ulf Ulmsten, the Swedish doctor who became known as the "father of TVT" (tension-free vaginal tape).

Ulmsten had decided to tackle an age-old female condition that in the modern age was ripe for a change. Ever since women have been having babies and growing older, they've been struggling with stress urinary incontinence (SUI) and pelvic organ prolapse (POP). Yet this female problem plagues half of the women over age 50—not just those who've had children.

Why does this happen?

SUI occurs when the muscles and tissues that support the bladder (pelvic floor muscles) and the muscles that regulate the release of urine (urinary sphincter) weaken usually due to childbearing or age (or both). When an activity like laughing or picking up something heavy puts force on the abdomen, pelvic area, or bladder, the weakened muscles can't keep the valve-like muscles in the urethra closed, so urine leaks out. No woman wants to leak pee and wear a pad all the time!

In the 1990s, colposuspension, or the "Burch procedure," was the go-to surgery for SUI. A surgeon would create an incision in the lower abdomen, and the urethra would be raised and held in place by stitches attached to ligaments at the back of the pubic bone. While this surgery was thought to be highly successful with two-thirds (66 percent) of women claiming they no longer had SUI, there was a long recovery time of three to four days in the hospital and approximately six weeks to fully heal. Due to the high cost, surgical invasiveness, and prolonged healing time, this option wasn't readily offered to women.

Then Ulmsten came onto the scene. In 1996, Ulmsten, an obstetrician and gynecologist at Uppsala University Hospital, Sweden's oldest university hospital, published a paper on the results of a new operation for female incontinence. Ulmsten and his colleagues had developed a procedure in which a surgeon inserted a narrow strip of plastic mesh tape to act as a hammock for the urethra. The tape was inserted through the vagina, threaded around the woman's urethra, and attached to her pubic bone. This revolutionary design, called tension-free vaginal tape, lets the bladder function normally in a woman until she has a sudden muscle contraction—from coughing, sneezing, or quickly changing her position. The contraction tightens the plastic hammock, which closes the opening of the urethra, keeping the bladder from releasing urine.

Ulmsten's paper, which appeared in March 1996 in the *International Urogynecology Journal*, reported that of 75 women who had undergone the procedure with him or members of his team, 63 patients—a whopping 84 percent—were "completely cured," according to a two-year follow-up. Another six of them were "significantly improved." Furthermore, this surgery was far less complex than the traditional incontinence surgery, the Burch method. It would only take about a half hour or less, and it could be performed under local anesthetic as an outpatient procedure.

"The financial implications were immediately obvious—especially to Ethicon," according to a lengthy investigation in the *British Medical Journal* in 2018. "Ethicon made Ulmsten an offer he couldn't refuse."

Ulmsten understood that his results might be considered, in his words, "too positive"—all 75 operations had been carried out by experienced urogynecologists in his department in their hospital. Ulmsten set out to organize a larger, multicenter study to find out how safe and effective this quick procedure could be in "ordinary" gynecological units.

Behind the scenes, Ulmsten had been asked by Ethicon to see if he could match the positive results of his first study. If a larger study could match or improve on those results, Ethicon would pay him $1 million to secure the rights to TVT, according to the *British Medical Journal*.

In February 1997, less than a year after the first study appeared, Ulmsten filed a US patent application naming himself and another colleague as the inventors. Ulmsten formed a company called Medscand to assign the patent and shortly afterward signed a licensing agreement with Johnson & Johnson (the parent company of Ethicon).

The results of Ulmsten's second study were even more positive than his first. The larger trial involved 131 women in six hospitals in Sweden and Finland. This time 91 percent—119 women—were "cured" after receiving the TVT implant, and another nine cases were "significantly improved." The study appeared in the *International Urogynecology Journal* in July 1998.

Ulmsten's million-dollar down payment multiplied. The *British Medical Journal* (*BMJ*) got Johnson & Johnson to confirm that in addition to the $1 million, the company had "paid Medscand a total of $24,525,000 in 1999 to purchase all assets associated with the TVT business."

Johnson & Johnson also acknowledged an important issue about timing to the *BMJ*. The company confirmed that "its lucrative financial offer to Ulmsten had been on the table before the second trial was carried out." However, J&J "rejected" any suggestion that the amount of money at stake had compromised the results of Ulmsten's trial.

This information wasn't well known within the urogynecological and ob-gyn community. Most doctors just knew that Ulmsten had become a consultant for J&J in the wake of those great results of the second bigger study.

The timing of Ulmsten's financial agreement with Ethicon didn't surface until 2014 in a lawsuit over damages to a mesh victim. During the trial, documents involving J&J and Dr. Ulmsten were shown to the jury, according to the *BMJ*.

> The message to Ulmsten implicit in the deal with Johnson & Johnson was "prove . . . that this procedure works and it is safe, and we'll pay you money . . . If you don't prove it, you don't get paid," Margolis said, according to *BMJ*. This was "wallet-driven research," he added.

Dr. Tom Margolis of California, a mesh removal specialist who was testifying for the plaintiff's side against Johnson & Johnson, was asked to give his opinion of the relationship between Ulmsten and Ethicon. Margolis calmly tore into their agreement. The message to Ulmsten implicit in the deal with Johnson & Johnson was "prove . . . that this procedure works and it is safe, and we'll pay you money . . . If you don't prove it, you don't get paid," Margolis said, according to *BMJ*. This was "wallet-driven research," he added.

And that is the tale of the big bang that gave the world vaginal mesh incontinence implants.

Johnson & Johnson kept Ulmsten busy. Around 1998, Ethicon sent a group of leading American urogynecologists to Sweden to learn the TVT implant procedure alongside Ulmsten and his team. Those American doctors became "preceptors" and KOLs (key opinion leaders) for Ethicon touting the virtues of vaginal mesh over the next several years.

Ulmsten worked with Ethicon's team as they updated versions of his basic TVT (transvaginal tape). But they still were not conducting real randomized clinical trials in women.

In fact, during one meeting of Ethicon's incontinence group in late 1999, Ulmsten discussed the kind of testing or studies that would be adequate for new TVT slings. The meeting minutes said, "Dr. Ulmsten was unclear how comparable the pig model was to humans, and assumed 5 to 10 pigs were sufficient for preclinical results."

Ulmsten's initial studies weren't just critical to the explosion of mesh products starting in the late 1990s. The only "long-term" studies of vaginal mesh in women were dependent on those studies and follow-up tests conducted by Ulmsten and later one of his colleagues, Carl Nilsson. That became the long-term "data" that industry waved around to fend off mounting complaints about mesh erosion and injuries. In 2018, Johnson & Johnson issued a statement through the Society of Urodynamics, Female Pelvic Medicine & Urogenital Reconstruction, defending studies that supported vaginal mesh implants. It said that in the 20 years since Ulmsten's first study, hundreds of other research trials "with no connection to Dr. Ulmsten or Ethicon" had validated the safety and effectiveness of pelvic mesh.

> The meeting minutes said, "Dr. Ulmsten was unclear how comparable the pig model was to humans, and assumed 5 to 10 pigs were sufficient for preclinical results."

Today, Ulmsten is revered in the medical community that treats women and their pelvic disorders. After his death in 2004, the International Urogynecological Association began hosting the Ulf Ulmsten Lecture at their annual meeting.

In 2014, the lecture was delivered by Carl Nilsson. His subject was "Creating a Gold Standard Surgical Procedure: The Development and

Implementation of TVT." Nilsson praised his late colleague Ulmsten during the talk. He reported on the long-term study of the safety and effectiveness of the TVT sling that had been updated several times since the early Ulmsten studies. Nilsson lauded the results of a 17-year review of the early TVT surgery patients, saying it showed that "no decline in cure rate has developed throughout the years and that no late onset problems occur with the polypropylene tape used in these by-now-rather-elderly women."

However, the *British Medical Journal* had a different view of the TVT's success rate, as seen in the follow-ups. In 2018, Carl Heneghan, editor of *BMJ*'s Evidence Based Medicine outlet, reviewed Nilsson's numbers. Heneghan noted that some medical publications were very impressed. "Here is what the Oxfordshire Clinical Commissioning Group reported: 'It confers a high prospect of long-term cure (published 17-year data shows 70–80 percent long-term efficacy) with a low risk of complication.'"

"Sounds good, doesn't it?" wrote Heneghan. Then he launched into his less positive analysis: "The original trial was done in three Nordic centres, and upon reading the trial publications closely (I found reports at 5, 7, 11 and 17 years of follow-up), what you find is a small study of 90 women and a denominator that shrinks over time . . . The shrinking denominator enhances the effect size and misleads the reader into thinking the effect is better than it actually is," Heneghan concluded.

What had happened was that after the original 90 women in the first trial, each follow-up study included fewer patients. That was due to deaths or the patients' inability to come to the study clinics for their evaluation. By the time of the last update, the study participants still reported overall satisfaction with their TVT implants and few complications, but by that time only about half the women were included. According to Heneghan, it's possible that only 47 percent of the women would be "cured."

If only researchers on both sides of this matter could look at the original Ulmsten study and follow-up data. Imagine them carefully reviewing various questions about "bias" in choice of patient or surgeon or hospital, and about the definition of "cured."

But that's not possible.

During various lawsuits and court hearings in recent years, it was revealed that some of the documentation relating to the early days of Ulmsten's company Medscand and TVT slings had been destroyed in a fire at a storage facility in Switzerland in 2009, according to the *British Medical Journal*. Destroyed documents included what one lawyer described as "the core Ulmsten data."

According to testimony in 2014, only a single binder of patient data from Ulmsten's multicenter study in Scandinavia survived.

From there, the use of transvaginal mesh snowballed and was marketed as the "gold standard" to address women's difficulties due to stress urinary incontinence.

THE NO-RULES RULE

To understand how Ulmsten's creation became both a blockbuster for sales and a disaster for many women, it's important to understand that, well—*it was the 1990s.* Or as some think of it, the era of regulatory free fall.

In 1993, Bill Clinton came to the White House, eager to prove that "moderate" Democrats like him and his vice president, Al Gore, could work with Republicans and Wall Street. It was time for government and the business sector to form partnerships—that's simply shorthand for deregulation.

While introducing plans to stimulate the economy, Clinton and Gore unveiled the National Partnership for Reinventing Government and the National Performance Review in 1993. The review of all the nation's agencies, including oversight divisions, would be based on "goals, not process"—in other words, on "measurements."

In early 1995, at a Reinventing Government event, Al Gore touted the arrival of "regulatory reform." He applauded the Performance Review's initial disposal of thousands of pages of "old-fashioned" rules and other impediments to America's business growth.

"We've been having numerous, very long nuts-and-bolts sessions ... And we've learned two basic practical lessons. First, we can cut back on the volume of regulations, and we are doing just that. Secondly, we can improve the relationship between regulators and the people they regulate. And when we do these things, we get better results for our country," he said.

"Business owners are sick of being treated like criminals. They see a government that just doesn't make sense, that charges them with safety violations when no one is in harm's way," Gore added.

So regulations were out and metrics were *in*. How many bank mergers did you approve? Hospital mergers? How much federal land did you open up for oil drilling? At the FDA, the ruling metric was very simple: How many drugs and medical devices did you approve this year?

> "Business owners are sick of being treated like criminals. They see a government that just doesn't make sense, that charges them with safety violations when no one is in harm's way," Gore added.

Finance, real estate, health care, energy—all the rules were loosened or dumped.

This was where the groundwork for the near-collapse of Wall Street and the housing industry in 2008—*The Big Short*—was laid.

As for the health-care industry, regulations involving everything from financial practices to safety standards practically disappeared. Because nature abhors a vacuum, big hospital systems took advantage of the lack of oversight to gouge and cheat insurers, patients, and the government. Doctors set records robbing from Medicare. Those frauds got the big headlines.

But the same behavior and the same complacency was at work less visibly in the pharmaceutical and medical device industries. Shielded by powerful lobbying groups, drug and device makers manipulated the system, cut corners, and downplayed or simply ignored terrible physical side effects linked to their products. Wall Street became enamored with the drug and device industries, and investors clamored for newer inventions and faster profits.

This period produced some of the worst decisions made by the Food and Drug Administration officials who approved pharmaceuticals and medical devices for sale in the US at an alarming rate—often over the objections of their own scientists inside the FDA who were worried about protecting the public.

There was a culture shift. The FDA began to refer to "stakeholders" in the system, which included companies. Patients were pushed further down the line of priorities.

In research, there were no concerns about "conflict of interest" when company-funded scientists published glowing studies about poorly tested drugs and devices. The top medical journals—*New England Journal of Medicine* and the *Journal of the American Medical Association*—did try to push back against shills for corporations and their ghostwritten reports. But that just prompted the creation of slews of niche medical journals that cranked out "peer-reviewed" articles night and day.

When patients suffered from terrible side effects—became ill or even died—drug and device makers and their lobbyists read from a well-rehearsed script: The companies were surprised, even shocked at the unexpected adverse effects. They had no warning their products were dangerous. These problems were all part of the cost of developing new and "innovative" treatments to give Americans the best health care in the world.

Then companies and their corporate defense attorneys would withdraw to restricted rooms stuffed with documents, where they tried to figure out how to guard themselves and their investors from memos, emails, and studies showing that they knew all along that their product was risky and that they had been playing with patients' lives.

"There really weren't many rules for device makers," said a former lobbyist for the medical device industry. "We'd beaten up the FDA so often, they didn't bother fighting us anymore."

"And Congress wasn't going to help," he added, laughing. Ironically, "some of the biggest consumer advocates in the Senate come from states with huge device makers like Medtronic." Politicians from

Massachusetts, Wisconsin, and Minnesota were not going to demand more control from the FDA over medical device companies.

It was during this time of the recession that Wall Street buzzed about the "female incontinence market" as prospectors once gushed about the California gold rush.

Women were changing, and so were their outlooks and opportunities: 60 was the new 40, and everyone was in aerobics classes or jogging or on the tennis court; they were becoming mothers later in life. It was much easier to stay younger longer.

> "There really weren't many rules for device makers," said a former lobbyist for the medical device industry. "We'd beaten up the FDA so often, they didn't bother fighting us anymore."

However, the pull of gravity did not care that you've come a long way, baby.

The evolution of the human body was still lagging behind at its own glacial pace. By 40, or after childbirth, or just because, parts of women's bodies were going to sag, starting with their breasts and genitalia.

Pelvic organ prolapse. Too much prolapse, and when you laughed or coughed or stood up to talk in a boardroom, you leaked a little. Playing sports such as tennis was a land mine for women—one jump or sudden stretch and it was time to go to the locker room and change pants.

It was embarrassing, and women rarely talked publicly about it.

But the medical industry and investors were already on it. Peeing unexpectedly was a "condition," and conditions need "treatments," and treatments need names. Stress urinary incontinence. SUI. Urethral hypermobility. Thanks to the increasing number of aging female baby boomers, the incontinence market had become the new frontier.

"This was a billion-dollar market, no question," said a longtime analyst on Wall Street who covers major medical device makers. "You've seen, it is much bigger than that now."

"Look, you had more women staying active longer, with jobs, aging baby boomers. The companies did not have to develop their market. The market for female incontinence products was growing itself!" the stock analyst added.

And so a horde of device makers rushed in, driven by the perspective that modern women, especially those with careers, didn't have time for Burch surgeries and hospital-bound recoveries. There had to be other ways to control leakage linked to pelvic organ prolapse. Boston Scientific, Johnson & Johnson's subsidiary Ethicon, American Medical Systems, C. R. Bard, Tyco, Coloplast, and others went to work.

WARNING SIGNS

During this time of deregulation and greed, the pharmaceutical companies found other areas where they could prey on women's insecurities and fight against the telltale signs of aging. A 2006 report called "The History of Drug Advertising: The Evolving Roles of Consumers and Consumer Protection" clearly explained, "in seeking to sell products, pharmaceutical marketers turn normal human experiences with things like hair loss or shyness into diseases." As appealing as a get-rich-quick scheme, doctors doled out medications promising miraculous results while ignoring to inform patients of any risks or side effects.

There were two easy, surefire ways to do this: through prescribing approved medications for "off-label" use, and by using the FDA's convenient loophole in the medical device application process called the 510(k) process.

Off-label use means that a drug (or medical device) can be mass-marketed for billions of dollars even though the FDA never approved it for that intended use. This is how it works: drug makers get their application approved for a narrow use in a small (maybe 100-person) group, obtain FDA approval, and then they put it on the market. By the time they are allowed to sell it, they've already done the numbers showing they can't make money just for this narrow purpose. But there's a secret plan in the works; the intended goal is to market it to as many people as they can to drive prescriptions for this miracle cure and make billions.

Technically, it's illegal to "market" a drug for off-label use. That's where company-funded medical studies come in handy—a sales rep can't suggest to a doctor to use a product off-label. But the rep can "educate" a doctor about medical research involving conditions that a specific drug or device could treat, which are not mentioned on the FDA-approved label.

> "Most people probably believe that when they get a medical device implanted, be it a pacemaker or a joint, that those medical devices have undergone appropriate testing to demonstrate that they are safe and effective before doctors started using them. But for most moderate and high-risk devices, that is not the case," states Dr. Michael Carome, director of Public Citizen's Health Research Group.

For medical products, the 510(k) process was originally designed to speed products to market to help those who desperately needed them. In the decades since, it has become the gaping loophole wherein a majority of devices are tossed to market with minimal human testing, which is expensive and time-consuming. A medical device company just needs to submit paperwork explaining that their new device has "substantial equivalence (SE) to a legally marketed (predicate) device. All 510(k)s provide a comparison between the device to be marketed and the predicate device or devices," explains the FDA.

"Most people probably believe that when they get a medical device implanted, be it a pacemaker or a joint, that those medical devices have undergone appropriate testing to demonstrate that they are safe and effective before doctors started using them. But for most moderate and high-risk devices, that is not the case," states Dr. Michael Carome, director of Public Citizen's Health Research Group.

But the dirty little secret of the FDA's Medical Devices division approval system is that, run by and for the industry, the agency OKs more than 90 percent of the products for sale through the weak and easily manipulated 510(k) process.

OVERUSE + OFF-LABEL USE = DISASTER

FEN-PHEN

This "miracle drug" combo was sold for obesity. The maker of one-half of that combination, dexfenfluramine, told the FDA when they approved it in 1996 that the company would only market its powerful new diet pill for the "morbidly obese."

But the drug, which instantly became a success, was mass-marketed as a way for women to quickly and easily lose five to 10 pounds. It was freely given out and nearly six million women took this pill for its tempting promise of weight loss. However, it was so strong that it was linked to permanent heart valve damage and to a lung condition, primary pulmonary hypertension, which was deadly in a number of women.

Dr. Michael Weintraub, a professor of clinical pharmacology at the University of Rochester, knew that fenfluramine and phentermine had been approved by the FDA decades earlier, so he had an idea to mix these two drugs together for off-label use. Dr. Weintraub tested the safety and effectiveness on a small study of just 12 participants (two-thirds were women) over four years. Since these individual drugs had been on the market for 10 and 12 years, he thought that all adverse effects were already known. However, when these two powerful drugs were used together, the FDA and doctors quickly saw an increase in the number of heart complications among women.

In May 1996, the FDA approved dexfenfluramine under its brand name, Redux. The next year, 291 patients, mostly women, had damaged heart valves. Ultimately, 175,000 claims were filed against the drug company. Redux was withdrawn from the market in September 1997.

VIOXX

Initially this popular drug was put on the market for arthritis, but Merck, its maker, encouraged its use for menstrual cramps and other common, painful conditions. To promote sales and expand the uses for Vioxx (Rofecoxib), a new study was performed to show that Vioxx had fewer gastrointestinal side effects than naproxen for the treatment of rheumatoid arthritis.

The results of this study were devastating to Merck: Vioxx was not only less effective in relieving symptoms of rheumatoid arthritis than naproxen but also proved to have an increased risk of myocardial infarction (heart attack). To scrub this report to make it palatable for approval, Merck tweaked the test time periods of the two drugs. They compared a shorter time period using Vioxx versus the adverse effects that occurred over a longer time in the naproxen group.

Merck sent this report to one million doctors and health professionals, boasting of the results, and even published their "findings" in credible medical journals including the *New England Journal of Medicine* and the *Annals of Internal Medicine*. Vioxx is said to have been linked to 60,000 deaths and was taken off the market in 2004.

So what do fen-phen and Vioxx have to do with pelvic mesh? They were all part of a commonly used practice called "off-label" use. Fen-phen was approved for obesity, Vioxx for arthritis, and plastic mesh for hernia repair.

However, these drugs and devices were over-marketed, lacked research, and harmed hundreds of thousands of patients since doctors didn't know the results of these time bombs in the human body. Lessons that could have been learned from the fen-phen and Vioxx scandals were quickly ignored.

FDA CHANGES SALES TACTICS

In 1938, Congress passed the Federal Food, Drug, and Cosmetic Act (FDCA) that for the first time required drugs to be proven safe and effective to receive approval from the FDA before they could be marketed and sold in the United States.

Included within the FDCA were new labeling requirements for drugs to ensure that consumers could understand the appropriate uses and directions on how to correctly use the medication. Additionally, these labeling requirements had to be placed on the package in a way that consumers would see it and be aware of its contents. Basically, they couldn't reduce it to tiny, unreadable print buried somewhere on an obscure location of the package.

"Between 1938 and 1951, federal drug legislation and regulation had a significant impact on the market for drugs, and between 1929 and 1949, the amount of money that consumers spent on drugs prescribed by doctors rose from 32 to 57 percent," explained Julie Donohue, author of the previously mentioned report, "A History of Drug Advertising." "By 1969, prescription drugs made up 83 percent of consumer spending on pharmaceuticals. Finally, between 1939 and 1959, drug sales rose from $300 million to $2.3 billion, with prescription drugs accounting for all but approximately $4 million of the increase."

With the end of World War II in 1945, self-medication in the United States was replaced by newer pharmacological treatments. Over time, many drugs previously made available for people to self-medicate with were available only through a doctor's prescription.

Shortly after these changes went into effect, the pharmaceutical industry realized it needed to abandon its direct-to-consumer advertising and focus all its advertising efforts directly toward physicians. Those in the industry realized that the physicians' "gatekeeper role" meant that they needed to sell the prescriptions and surgical implants to the physicians so they would then sell them to their patients. "By the 1960s more than 90 percent of the pharmaceutical companies' spending on marketing was aimed at doctors (with the rest targeting pharmacists and hospitals)," Donohue states. This was "a complete reversal of the pattern thirty years earlier."

While looking at this brief history about how the FDA came to be and how pharmaceutical companies established their marketing practices, it's important to note that the regulations that were enforced were primarily focused on drugs, not devices. The 1920s, '30s, and '40s had a saturated market full of phony gadgets promoted with outlandish promises like orbs that generated "z-rays" to cure arthritis and vibrating belts that melted away belly fat. Device regulation didn't come into play until 1976, when the FDA stepped in to attempt to monitor what doctors were using on and in their patients' bodies.

By then, regulators were too late and too lax. The medical device industry quickly became known as the "Wild West" of medicine—the applications of rules and regulations were haphazard. The medical device industry learned the fine art of lobbying in Washington and turned it into a science.

In the popular Netflix documentary *The Bleeding Edge*, Dr. David Kessler, FDA commissioner from 1990 to 1997, states that "we built a system that doesn't work." True, it's one where marketing has become more influential than medicine.

In fact, nearly 70 million people have had medical device implants put in them within the past 10 years and 98 percent of those were fast-tracked through the previously mentioned 510(k) process. Only 2 percent go through the premarket approval process, which means being tested in a human before being put on the market.

The tragedy of transvaginal mesh didn't occur overnight. Many factors had to come together in a perfect storm to create an environment of complacency, blind faith in medicine, industry loopholes, and marketing over morals. All this allowed companies to market to the modern woman by implying that her worth was inextricably tied to her youth.

CHAPTER 3

WALLET-DRIVEN MISSION

What is the real percentage of adverse events from the product? "We reviewing 99 patients and observed a 30% complication rate."

—Boston Scientific memo, April 1999, on talking points to explain at medical convention why ProtoGen was recalled

"Whenever doctors say 'the majority of women to undergo mesh procedures were not harmed, etc . . .' they are just trying to deflect attention away from the medical profession's blame in the mesh scandal. Remember Thalidomide—the popular insomnia drug for pregnant women which caused thousands of severe birth defects in the 1960s? No one said, 'Oh yes, but hundreds of thousands of women got a good night's sleep on Thalidomide, and that outweighs the harm.'"

—Danny Vadasz, CEO of the Health Issues Centre in Australia, The Guardian 2017

No one agrees exactly when the 25-year scandal over vaginal mesh began, but almost everyone agrees that it could have been avoided.

And there's no better example of this than the miserable tale of the first product marketed that flung the doors open for various versions of vaginal mesh: ProteGen.

Boston Scientific had been on a buying spree in the mid-1990s to vacuum up smaller companies with innovative devices. The company was determined to corner a major piece of the SUI business. It planned to market a device that would replace the then-accepted surgery for incontinence, the hour-long "Burch procedure," which required slicing open the abdomen to get to the pelvic area and keeping the patient in the hospital for a couple of days.

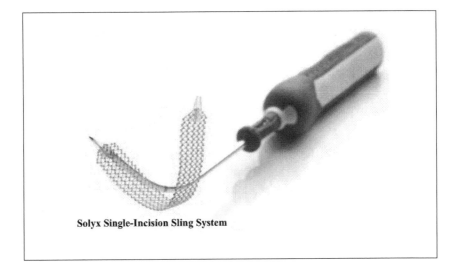

Solyx Single-Incision Sling System

Instead, Boston Scientific would use a shortcut—the vagina—to reach the pelvic bone, where they would nail two pins to which they would attach a sort of hammock (a narrow sling), to support the urethra. That would keep the bladder from pressing too much on the urethra and limit those sudden SUI moments. The operation would take only 30 minutes, and the patient could probably go home that very day. It was revolutionary. The scientific thinking was: If a piece of plastic mesh could be safely put into a man's wide midriff to close a hole in the abdominal wall or a muscle, why wouldn't the same mesh work when pushed into a tight area containing women's reproductive organs?

Boston Scientific knew it was not the only medical device maker with the vaginal passage idea. But it hoped to be the first to sell such a sling, with the appropriate instruments and pins that would form a package. During its acquisition spree it had bought a San Clemente company called Vesica Medical that made a device that could pin two hangers on the pelvic bone, called the Vesica Bone Anchoring System. Intended for urinary incontinence, the Vesica system was not inserted transvaginally.

But Boston Scientific was developing the hammock sling to implant through the vagina and attach to the pelvic bone. Boston Scientific would sell the two products together, the Vesica anchors and the ProteGen Sling as a "kit."

And that is how ProteGen became the first major disaster in the new world of pelvic mesh.

ProteGen was launched with a lot of publicity in 1997 and formally recalled in early 1999. It set in motion a series of predictable (and predicted) mistakes, shortcuts, and mix-ups that put millions of women's lives at risk all for the sake of greed.

But before Boston Scientific even made this first version of the ProteGen Sling, there are several glaring obstacles that would shoot down the theory that mesh in the vagina was a good idea in the mind of any competent doctor.

First of all, plastic mesh wasn't tested in women's vaginas before it was sold, so neither the amount of mesh nor the kind of plastic used was studied in clinical trials. To get away with this, mesh makers abused a huge loophole in FDA regulations—a loophole rabidly guarded by the medical device lobby. The 510(k) process, as mentioned earlier, allows companies a relative "pass" from federal regulators if their product is remotely similar to any other product (in this case, plastic hernia mesh) that has been tested and is on the market, no matter how long ago that earlier product was approved.

However, even Boston Scientific's own leadership knew that medical devices should be tested in humans first—just not live ones. In a 2015 testimony, Alfred Intoccia Jr., who was the research and development director for the Urology and Women's Health division at Boston Scientific in 2001, was asked if products should be tested in the area where the device will be used. He replied, "Absolutely. It's called design validation . . . We did many, many, many cadaver labs. So they were placed in the female vagina by physicians, and we learned a tremendous amount from that approach."

So while Intoccia admitted that products need to be tested, mesh kits were only placed in cadavers, which wouldn't show the long-term effects of mesh shrinkage, migration, pain during sex, inability to have children, and other complications that a living subject would be forced to endure. It's like putting a new form of fuel in a car and never driving it. Of course no adverse results are apparent because it's at rest, but once the engine is turned on and the car comes to life, the true results become evident.

> "Be first to market—time to market is the most critical measure of long-term business success when developing a new product."

Unfortunately, Boston Scientific felt that time was not on their side and actual clinical testing of their nascent mesh product would take too long. In the same deposition cited above, Intoccia read notes from a R&D Department meeting from October 2004 that stated, "Be first to market—time to market is the most critical measure of long-term business success when developing a new product." Not patient health, not product safety, but "time to market" paired with "long-term business success."

It gets worse. Not only had the mesh implant not been tested in the vaginas of live women, but the surgical procedure to implant the new incontinence slings hadn't been tested either.

This is where Newton's law of gravity would have come in handy.

It is easier to lift organs from above than to push them upward from below. As Sir Isaac Newton said of gravity, "What goes up must come down."

But the new mesh implants, designed to replace the cumbersome Burch procedure, involved going into a body cavity underneath the drooping organs by making incisions through the vagina—where you cannot see. Why not go in through a laparoscopy, aided by microscopic cameras, and raise up the organs to position them? "Everybody knows it's better to go down through the abdominal area," a salesman who handled prolapse mesh and incontinence slings said several times during interviews. "The doctors all knew that."

Here's another issue that earlier clinical testing might have helped. The vagina itself can never be completely sterile and provides a different environment for mesh (as compared to the abdomen and the use of hernia mesh).

Infection is a real, not a rare, risk. According to Dr. Donald Ostergard, an obstetrician-gynecologist, "The vagina is a clean-contaminated environment, and it is not possible to insert polypropylene mesh devices without bacterial contamination, despite standard antibiotic usage. Once inserted, the host tissue immediately attaches to the polypropylene and attempts to defend it from bacterial invasion, but if the bacteria have already reached the surface of the device, then dislodgement is difficult. The devices with larger surface areas result in greater bacterial contamination, more polypropylene degradation, increased inflammatory response, fibrous tissue stimulation, and erosion."

And here's the last general issue that should have been a red flag. *There was no exit strategy, no plan B, no way to get the mesh out.*

At this time, polypropylene mesh had been used for hernia surgery for over three decades. The point of mesh to repair hernias is to reinforce and support the torn tissue. The mesh is placed inside the abdomen, where tissue grows in and around the device. However, hernia mesh surgeries are far from problem-free. Many times the body rejects the foreign implant, which results in inflammation and biocompatibility issues. It was already well known that hernia mesh can result in hernia recurrence, infection, and adhesions (when scar tissue forms around the mesh implant and joins the implant with other internal tissue or organs, causing immense pain and discomfort). Additionally, once tissue forms in and around the mesh, it can be quite complicated—if not impossible—to remove the entire device from the body. (With TVM, the doctors and researchers were focused on putting it in quickly without considering how it could be taken out. This will become a devastating issue.)

Mesh survivor Tammy Jackson was featured on *The Bleeding Edge*, where she told her heartbreaking story. She noticed that after having her daughter, she would leak urine when she would attempt to move a patient during her job as a pediatric nurse. At her doctor's visit, he promised her that this quick 45-minute procedure involving mesh would easily solve her problem. After the surgery, she felt terrible pain, was vomiting, and had a terrible fever. After several ER and doctor visits, one doctor finally determined it was the mesh that was causing her sickness. Tammy recalls, "He said, 'You've got a problem with your mesh. It needs to be removed, but I can't do it. I've never been trained to take it out. I've never taken it out. We were just trained on how to put it in.'"

> "You've got a problem with your mesh. It needs to be removed, but I can't do it. I've never been trained to take it out. I've never taken it out. We were just trained on how to put it in."

"I've had major surgery: bladder repair, cervix removal, reconstruction," Tammy says. She's had 18 surgeries and has not been able to have sex with her husband for eight years.

But none of these three major issues stopped mesh makers from their pursuit of market share and profits. During the height of the vaginal mesh craze in the US, roughly 1999–2012, corporations made billions of dollars in revenues.

Doctors, thanks to the embrace of prolapse mesh kits and incontinence slings by their esteemed medical associations—the American College of Obstetricians and Gynecologists and the American

Urogynecologic Society—made millions. So did hospitals who shared in kickbacks from their exclusivity contracts with specific mesh makers.

Politicians were rewarded with millions in campaign donations from medical device makers determined to maintain their stranglehold on the FDA's lax medical device approval system and its invaluable loophole.

The only people who didn't get rich from the mesh scheme were the women, who were left for roadkill.

MESH MANIPULATION

There were many reasons why pelvic mesh wasn't a good idea, and more reasons would surface over the years. However, in 1995, Boston Scientific was focused on only four complications they had to overcome. The potential problems with its female sling program were laid out in an August 15, 1995, memo:

- Infection—The physicians are deeply concerned about the effect of infection of the urethra and pelvic bone. This concern appears to be coupled with use of synthetic materials passing from the vaginal canal into the abdominal area, which can provide a haven for colonizing bacteria.
- Erosion—This can occur from mechanical sawing of the urethra by a "rasp-like" sling material or an undetected bacterial infection.
- Surgical technique—The current technique of dissecting the interstitial tissue between the urethra and upper vaginal wall may be extremely difficult in some patients and require considerable surgical skill.
- Bladder dysfunction—Over-tensioning of the sling may result in the patient placed in permanent retention.

In hindsight, Boston Scientific's foresight was remarkable. Those were exactly the top four problems that later caused serious, often permanent physical damage in tens of thousands of women with vaginal mesh implants.

Unfortunately, Boston Scientific was long on discussion and short on fixes.

Six months later, on January 8, 1996, Boston Scientific's incontinence advisory committee met and discussed various incontinence-related projects at Boston Scientific and elsewhere. Bill Martin, who was ProteGen's product manager, wrote positively about the board's outreach to more physicians who might use and talk about Boston Scientific incontinence products.

He never mentioned "ProteGen" in the memo, but it hovered over all three pages.

Martin raised the plan for the upcoming convention of the American Urological Association (AUA), where Boston Scientific might mention its developmental "vaginal wall sling." "General consensus was reached that our focus for the AUA '96 should be introducing the concept of incorporating bone anchoring into various sling techniques rather than advocating only one approach (in situ vaginal wall)," wrote Martin. In other words, go gently, gently; don't blast it out. Surgeons don't like to be pressured into major changes to the way they operate, so to speak.

"Current thinking is that this might best be accomplished via training materials to be distributed at the AUA." This, added Martin, would "lay solid groundwork for future developments in the sling arena," for example, ProteGen.

Further on in that memo, one of Boston Scientific's consulting thought leaders, Dr. Rodney Appell, a longtime urologist who was researching new ways to address incontinence, raised concerns about potential erosion and infection with synthetic mesh proposed for a new Boston Scientific sling. Appell and two other doctors at the meeting indicated that "due to the sketchy history of synthetics, animal data is mandatory before we give it serious consideration."

There were also clinical and mechanical concerns about the unusual transvaginal approach to the implant. The "mushy" pelvic bone might not hold the mesh anchors, and there were infection concerns "due to the direct path from vagina to bone," participants said.

The memo ended, "Dr. Appell suggested a cautious approach to this technology until some of these questions are resolved."

Apparently, there was little interest in a cautious approach. By the first week of March, Bill Martin was exuberantly touting the lucrative future of ProteGen. "We project that 35,000+ of these procedures will be performed in 1997, with that number growing to 55,000 within 5 years," he wrote in a memo.

"We anticipate our first-year volume to be at least 5,000 units," with growth anticipated between 80 and 100 percent per year for at least the first five years, Martin continued. "We need to continue moving quickly and steadily on this project so we can begin realizing our market potential very soon."

> **"We need to continue moving quickly and steadily on this project so we can begin realizing our market potential very soon."**

Boston Scientific pushed its ProteGen forward to the FDA for expedited approval to market. Actually, Boston Scientific didn't apply for "approval," but for the notorious and easier 510(k) "clearance." That was because, according to Boston Scientific documents, ProteGen was similar to other devices on the market that were also constructed of Mersilene mesh, a popular mesh patch used in thousands of hernia surgeries. ProteGen's mesh was also successfully used in cardiovascular graft procedures.

Let's pause here. Hernia mesh was a thick, somewhat dense plastic mesh that seemed to function very well when placed flat in a person's abdomen; it covered weaknesses or small tears (hernias) in the intestines and muscles.

But the vaginal and pelvic areas aren't flat. They're delicate and home to major organs and blood vessels.

Furthermore, this mesh had not been tested in urological clinical studies. It certainly had not been tested in a vagina—unless you counted the vaginas of large dogs used in early vaginal mesh trials in Sweden for another kind of implant.

The mesh had, however, been tested in living beings—specifically 90 rats.

Remember, in the United States, medical devices could be "cleared" for sale if they were in some way "substantially equivalent" to other devices that at some point in history had actually been approved. Any attempt to force device makers to conduct clinical trials on "equivalent" devices was denounced as a return to the regulatory hell that Clinton and Gore had sworn to end.

Hernia mesh had been approved in the 1970s, and by around 1990, mesh accounted for nearly 90 percent of hernia repairs. This new vaginal mesh was related to that much older hernia repair material in that they were both knitted plastic, and under the lax law governing medical devices that was "close enough."

A "clearance," the FDA has stressed, does not mean the device is considered effective and safe; it means only that it is similar to another device already on the market.

ProteGen's mesh called Hemashield was made of Dacron, a form of polyester, and it was coated in bovine collagen, which experts said would enhance growth in patients' scar tissue around and through the pores in the mesh, covering and securing it.

The ProteGen Sling was cleared by the FDA in late 1996, and Boston Scientific began marketing it in early 1997. Bill Martin, ProteGen's product manager, moved pieces around for the launch strategy, nudging Boston Scientific to focus on the likely customers, urogynecologists, and their upcoming annual convention.

"As you are aware, each day prior to the April 11 AUA convention that these products are available in the marketplace is of significant, exponential value to Boston Scientific strategically as well as financially," wrote Martin on March 7, 1997.

Sure enough, in the first two months ProteGen was on the market, Boston Scientific sold almost $1 million worth of the slings.

CA-SLING!

But almost as soon as that number was reached, Boston Scientific started receiving complaints about problems involving ProteGen. In its first nine months on sale, ProteGen sparked 56 serious "adverse event" notices to the Food and Drug Administration.

And there were more issues. During a November 1997 meeting of Boston Scientific's new Incontinence Team, company medical experts raised concerns about ProteGen's biocompatibility in patients. The sling did not appear to promote the "scar-tissue-in-growth" that company representatives and medical spokespeople had described to urologists and pelvic surgeons and that its marketing materials had touted. It seemed that some patients' tissue cells were "rejecting" the mesh. That was particularly surprising, because, after all, the mesh was coated in collagen to enhance tissue formation.

Over the next six months, ProteGen sales continued to spike. So did adverse event reports—another 57 reached the FDA, bringing the total of adverse drug events to 113. At this point, people at Boston Scientific and at the Food and Drug Administration had to know they were in the middle of a health-care disaster involving a wildly popular product—so popular, in fact, that other companies were moving faster to get their own mesh slings to market to compete with ProteGen.

In fact, they did know. One lengthy memo said, with no irony, "In hindsight, to launch ProteGen, [Boston Scientific] needed greater understanding of ProteGen risks." The memo was dated April 20, 1998. The memo reflected marketing division interviews with 12 Boston Scientific sales reps who were promoting ProteGen to doctors and were facing resistance among their medical clientele. Though the rate of complications was "average," about 5 percent, the memo said, the rate of dissatisfied MDs was 18 percent. Close to a third of the doctors who had implanted ProteGen regularly did not intend to use it again. Its most common "complication" was dehiscence, a catchall term for a surgical incision reopening. The mesh was eroding in women and poking through their vaginal walls and slicing into their bladders and urethras.

Although surgical "technique" was thought to be the reason for most complications, the sales reps said some serious damage was reported in sling patients even when the surgeons had followed company instructions carefully and had gained experience doing several implantations. Then the memo laid out the wider landscape. "There is general concern amongst Reps regarding ongoing ProteGen complications and impact on overall business/company image," it read.

What's more, the rate of complications was higher than anticipated (and perhaps higher than what was being reported). "There currently is confusion and concern in the Field due to conjecture of true complication rates and impressions that complications (in particular, dehiscence) will continue. This situation sets a stage for unwanted rumors which may damage [Boston Scientific] Urology's image." At one point the memo indicated that Boston Scientific reps felt the company's message should "reposition expectation of complication rates."

The news became bleaker. Boston Scientific didn't have enough "champions" and "well-known thought leaders" who did ProteGen implants as the primary procedure for incontinence.

Additionally, one of the company's outside "champions," a leading physician, was "delivering unfavorable messages to other MDs." One rep said the former Boston Scientific fan was "poisoning our reputation."

The lack of supportive "champions" for Boston Scientific wouldn't have worried patients. But the reps' reports on the ProteGen surgery training system would have, and might have driven patients away—if they knew about it.

"Reps primarily trained MDs on ProteGen," the memo said. "Preceptors were rarely used," it added, referring to urologists experienced in incontinence surgery who, it was hoped, would proctor doctors who were starting ProteGen implants.

"ProteGen required a different sales approach (changing a technique vs. selling commonly accepted products) and comprehensive surgical knowledge," said the memo's findings. "Additionally, this product introduction occurred at a time when a lot of Reps were relatively new."

"If we had more training, we wouldn't be backpedaling now," one sales rep had commented.

Another rep unfavorably compared Boston Scientific's approach to Johnson & Johnson's, saying, "At Ethicon, we trained on animals; we understood tissue layers and had total appreciation of anatomy."

Were Boston Scientific's sales reps prepared to tell surgeons where to put an incision in the vagina and how to place the mesh? Not all of them thought so.

But the sales rep review was not the only memo bobbing around Boston Scientific that spring. The Boston Scientific Incontinence Team held its monthly meeting on April 10, where doctors and others raised questions about the mesh material itself. They also debated what to do with significant differences in the numbers and therefore the rate of complications among ProteGen patients.

To help limit possible damage from ProteGen, the mesh design needed to be modified. It "needs to be more porous to foster more ingrowth. The holes on the side could also be larger," the memo said team members indicated.

Varying skills (or lack of them) among surgeons implanting ProteGen was another issue affecting the sling's success. Dr. Appell, the urologist, suggested utilizing animation to help train doctors to implant the mesh.

The team discussed the continuing concerns with the sling's "limited clinical data." The memo noted that Dr. Appell's "thoughts on this area are well known."

But another consulting urologist present for the meeting dismissed the ongoing worries about the uncertain number of "complications" linked to ProteGen. The physician said that Boston Scientific "needs to get over the ProteGen issue.

"It is a good product, but it is a synthetic and will experience some complications," like all such synthetics. He said the company needed to "come up with a consistent message on the ProteGen complication rate.

"Boston Scientific should move on to something else," he suggested.

The group scheduled the next meeting of the Incontinence Team for May 14, and that was that.

To: File

From: Bill Martin

Date: January 8, 1996

Re: *Incontinence Advisory Board Meeting, January 7, 1996*

This note serves to summarize key thoughts and idea exchanges which resulted from our recent incontinence advisory board meeting. Overall, the meeting was a success, accomplishing our key objectives of: establishing our "new" relationship with these physicians; facilitating a healthy exchange of ideas; affirming our strategic directions; and exposing these physicians to the board array of resources at BSC. Key takeaways are as follows:

I.   *Multicenter Data-* It was quickly identified that we are missing some major patient numbers in our data. Now that collection of this data is being controlled by Dan Stoutenburgh, we should expect a radical improvement in the accuracy of the data. Additionally, Dan is aggressively looking to hire additional support for collection and management of this outcomes data.

II.   *Vaginal Wall Sling-* General consequences was reached that our focus for the AUA 96 should be introducing the concept of incorporating bone anchoring into various sling techniques rather than advocating only one approach (in-stiuvaginal wall). Current thinking is that this might best be accomplished via training materials to be distributed at the AUA. This would compliment several papers which would also be presented at the meeting and lay solid groundwork for future developments in the sling arena.

III. *Percutaneous Sling-* Current thinking is that our initial product should focus on simplifying the existing technique of sling surgery and we needn't be concerned about what type of vaginal incision a physician chooses to make. All three physicians confirm that anything which simplifies this very technically challenging procedure should be well accepted.

A. **Material Types**

      1. *Organogenesis*- This potentially holds some promise but at this point is still way off the mark in terms of availability and cost.

      2. *Human Tissue*- Group consensus was that we should categorically eliminate the consideration of any human tissue due to concerns about rejection, supply, and disease transmission.

      3. *Animal Tissue*- Bovine Pericardium has currently emerged as the leading candidate of all natural materials. Biovascualr offers a significant advantage to us in that they currently hold 510K approval, however, the physicians placed no value on the unique Tissue Guard processing which results in lower residual glutaraldehyde levels. They stated that this was potentially a significant advantage for the vascular system, but was insignificant for use in soft tissue placement.

      4. *Synthetics*- Primary concerns regarding synthesis were confirmed as erosion and infection. Dr. Appell stated that in looking at these two, his belief was that the erosion was caused by a combination of infection and pressure resulting from improper tensioning. Therefore, given that his belief was that infection issues related to synthetics were rotes in the growth of bacteria within the interstices present in synthetic materials. This could indicate that coated synthetic materials hold promise. All three doctors indicated that due to the sketchy history of synthetics, animal data is mandatory before we give it serious consideration.

IV. *Transvaginal Approach*- Although this approach sounds good conceptually, there were several clinical and mechanical concerns which were raised.

      A. Based on the study of 10+ cadavers, the consistency of the underside of the human pelvic bone is mushy, almost like styrofoam. This creates doubt as to the ability to securely attach an anchor to this position.

      B. Infection concerns due to the direct path from vagina to bone.

C. Questions as to whether a broad support of tissue could be achieved from one or two anchor points in such close proximity to the vaginal tissue.

D. Dr. Appell suggested a cautious approach to this technology until some of these questions are resolved.

THE FDA DRINKIN' THE KOOL-AID . . . AGAIN

Between the mounting pile of adverse event reports at the FDA and the barrage of complaints from doctors, both the government and Boston Scientific should have been well aware of the threats ProteGen posed. But what they knew and what they did about it were completely different things. This is where the ProteGen story becomes outrageous.

In June 1998, FDA officials visited a Boston Scientific plant and learned that the ProteGen problem was worse than they'd been informed. "During the inspection, it was learned that the number of events being reported is approximately two-thirds of the complaints being made to the firm," the FDA said. The FDA noted that the company had reported cases in which the device had to be surgically removed, according to a Newark *Star-Ledger* story from 1999.

There was more: 12 days before the agency inspection, Boston Scientific learned of at least 233 other cases with medical complications, according to a company document cited by the *Star-Ledger*.

"There are many patients with exposed slings that have not yet become symptomatic," the Boston Scientific memo said. "There is a large pool of patients entering the 4- to 9-month complication range that could present." A large pool indeed; by this time, Boston Scientific had sold at least 10,000 ProteGen/Vesica kits.

The company's memo suggested that the complications with ProteGen were not caused by the product, but the doctors' poor surgical techniques and poor choice of patients.

True to form, the FDA did not overreact. In its inspection report dated August 18, 1998, it said that "Boston Scientific is not involved in any activities at the present time that could be considered to be a recall."

"They have not issued any advisory notices to their customers that might be considered as being of the nature of a safety alert," the report said. "At the present time the rate of complaints appears to still be increasing for this device."

The government indicated that it was concerned that Boston Scientific was not being particularly responsive, but it took no action to halt sales or warn the public. Doctors continued implanting the sling.

Six months later, on January 22, 1999, Boston Scientific announced it would recall the device. By that time, it had been implanted in some 17,000 women.

ProteGen "does not produce outcomes that are consistent with the company's standard of performance for its products or customer expectations," said the company's official announcement. "The use of the ProteGen in the treatment of female urinary incontinence is associated with a higher rate than expected of vaginal erosion and dehiscence."

The FDA statement called the device "misbranded and adulterated," and said it "does not appear to function as intended."

ProteGen, Boston Scientific's answer to female incontinence, had been on the market less than two years.

THE PROTEGEN AUTOPSY

What went wrong? Almost everything.

First, the need to be first to market with a "sling kit" led to a series of bad decisions.

Boston Scientific encountered manufacturing issues after ProteGen was cleared in late 1996. That pushed back ProteGen's move to market, which in turn upset the revenue model.

To address the financial effects of that delay, Boston Scientific decided to skip its original plan to initially provide the sling to a select group of doctors so they could monitor its performance before its widespread distribution. Instead, propelled by the "rush to market," ProteGen made a big splash at the urologists' convention and sales just took off.

Next, the collagen-coated mesh had not been tested in women's pelvic areas. Boston Scientific was told in a consultant's report that the complication rate for ProteGen was higher than other implant materials. The report stated that woven polyester coated with bovine collagen could not be ruled out as a cause. Eventually, scientists became concerned that the collagen was preventing tissue cells from growing around and through the mesh, almost guaranteeing quick erosion and shrinkage of the sling.

But collagen wasn't necessarily the only issue with the mesh. In April 1998, Boston Scientific's Incontinence Team had acknowledged that the mesh should be "more porous to foster more ingrowth. The holes on the side could also be larger."

Luckily for Boston Scientific, by March it was already working to replace ProteGen with a successor product, the ProteGen II. They had quietly decided to continue selling the original ProteGen until it developed the successor sling, according to court documents.

A new version of the sling, of course, would do nothing for women who had already been implanted with ProteGen's early defective mesh, or for those who would be implanted before ProteGen II made its big entrance. As a later study in the *American Journal of Obstetrics and Gynecology* punned, those women were "left to their own devices."

Then, there was the big-picture issue with the mesh. For a device to be biocompatible with the human body, it must not only be well tolerated in the body generally but must function well in the particular body part where it will be implanted.

The Dacron collagen-coated mesh had never been tested in urological studies in a human and never in a woman's pelvis. No wonder that, among other things, Boston Scientific reps were getting complaints from surgeons that the mesh would not lie flat and tended to bunch up or that scar tissue wasn't growing quickly and smoothly over the implant.

What else? Some adverse event reports said mesh implants had to be removed from patients months after the surgery. However, the company didn't publicly acknowledge or warn patients about the radical nature of that resolution.

Because mesh was supposed to be a permanent implant, the companies had not planned for "removal." There were no instructions on how to do that, no surgeons trained in removing the mesh. It is a risky, complex procedure, and unlike the implant, the explant isn't a 30-minute process; it can take several hours and usually requires anesthesia.

Many women suffering from eroded mesh could not get their physicians to take their complaints about searing pain seriously. Instead, a number were told by their doctors that they were suffering from depression or fibromyalgia and to see pain management specialists or physical therapists. They were told that their problems were in their heads, not their vaginas. They were sent to psychiatrists.

> Many women suffering from eroded mesh could not get their physicians to take their complaints about searing pain seriously. They were told that their problems were in their heads, not their vaginas. They were sent to psychiatrists.

"After two visits back to my doctor, he told me I needed to go to a counselor," said a woman from the Philadelphia area who had the ProteGen implant. "I had to fly to California to get it removed," she added. "And I'm still in pain."

Finally, although Boston Scientific's embarrassing recall was a red flag to regulators, the ProteGen disaster did not promote action at the FDA or changes to the agency's medical device expedited-approval-and-clearance process.

PICKING UP THE PIECES

In April 1999, the annual AUA urologists' convention was coming up. However, this time, Boston Scientific's people weren't rolling out ProteGen; they were trying to explain it.

An internal memo proposed talking points for those attending the conference. One said that the types of clinical complications observed in ProteGen were similar to those seen in studies of other synthetic sling materials. However, "the rate of vaginal erosion was higher than our acceptable standard of performance."

The memo also laid out a sample Q&A script to follow when talking to AUA members or convention groups about ProteGen:

Why did you launch ProteGen and keep it on the market?

"Prior to its release, the product met all of the standard engineering and biocompatibility testing commonly applied to implants and it satisfied all US and European regulatory requirements."

The sample answer didn't mention that ProteGen didn't have clinical trials in women, that the testing involved rats, and that the product started out as a hernia mesh.

What should I tell my patients that underwent the ProteGen Sling procedure?

"The recall does not apply to products already implanted in patients."

What do I say to my patients who are threatening to sue?

"This product was cleared with the FDA and properly launched in the marketplace as a device for this indication."

ProteGen "responders" attending AUA were prepped to prepare for tough questions about the sling's alarming rates of side effects.

Is it true that adverse events with ProteGen are dramatically higher than you originally anticipated?

"The results are higher than anticipated. We have observed a high variance in procedural outcomes."

What is the real percentage of adverse events from the product?

"We reviewed 99 patients and observed a 30% complication rate."

Why are these numbers so much higher than other sling procedures?

"Bruce, David," began the answer, calling to Boston Scientific executives further up the food chain for help. "How do we answer this question?"

The memo became one of several times in the post-ProteGen review that Boston Scientific pledged to change its ways.

"In connection with any future sling materials, Boston Scientific will gather clinical data to assess product performance in a broad spec-

> Yes, you can use a medical device that has been recalled as the standard for expedited clearance with the Food and Drug Administration.

trum of clinical situations."

ProteGen was officially defunct. But like those scary movies where the dead villain springs back up, ProteGen still had life in it. Because even while the FDA and Boston Scientific were investigating all the injuries linked to ProteGen, other companies were citing ProteGen as their new mesh devices' "substantially equivalent" predicate.

Yes, you can use a medical device that has been recalled as the standard for expedited clearance with the Food and Drug Administration. That's how Johnson & Johnson's Gynecare TVT (tension-free vaginal tape) line and a dozen mesh devices made by American Medical Systems, Tyco, and others would get to market over the next five years.

"It defies logic," says Suzanne, who was treated with Ethicon's (Johnson & Johnson) transvaginal (tension-free) surgical mesh, which was predicated on the Boston Scientific ProteGen Sling. "Common sense should have dictated that all devices that had received approval using the ProteGen Sling as their predicate device would have also been pulled from the market."

"It's not a regulatory requirement to do so," says Siobhan DeLancey, press officer for the Center for Devices and Radiological Health to *IB News.* "We have an informal policy, if the predicate was withdrawn because of manufacturing, not specifications itself, then we may not look at a 510(k) device. It's kind of a case-by-case basis."

Although ProteGen may have been taken off the market, the door was now forced wide open for other mesh products to enter the market—based on the disgraced ProteGen—to become highly profitable at the cost of women's health.

And so, ProteGen was not only the predicate for many other devices but became the template for the entire mesh scandal.

Almost all the poor decisions that were made during ProteGen's brief existence were about to be repeated. And repeated. And repeated.

D. Chart of Boston Scientific's Transvaginal Mesh Kits Released Through the 510 (k) process

TIMELINE OF REGULATORY EVENTS

YEAR	DATE	ACTION	DEVICE(S)
2002	January 9th	k020110-510(k) Submission	Advantage, Advantage Fit and Lynx
	April 3rd	K020110-510(k) Clearance	Advantage, Advantage Fit and Lynx
	August 23rd	Limited Launch	Advantage and Lynx
2003	December 5th	Full Launch	Advantage and Lynx
2004	March 26th	K040787-510(k) Submission	Prefyx and Obtryx
	April 14th	K040787-510(k) Clearance	Prefyx and Obtryx
	August 12th	Launch	Obtryx
2007	Febuary 15th	Launch	Prefyx
	July 12th	K0719570-510(k) Submission	Pinnacle
	November 8th	K0719570-510(k) Clearance	Pinnacle
2008	January 21st	Launch	Pinnacle
	April 11th	K081048- 510(k) Submission	Uphold
	April 18th	Launch	Advantage Fit
	May 2nd	K081275-510(k) Submission	Solyx
	August 22nd	K081048- 510(k) Clearance	Uphold
	August 27th	K081275-510(k) Clearance	Solyx
	October 13th	Launch	Uphold
	December 5th	Launch	Solyx
2009	April 19th	K091131-510(k) Submission	Pinnacle Duet
	May 12th	K091131-510(k) Clearance	Pinnacle Duet
	November 13th	Launch	Pinnacle Duet
2010	November 22nd	K103426-510(k) Submission	LITE PFR Kits
2011	September 14th	K103426-510(k) Clearance	LITE PFR Kits
2012	January 3rd	FDA Orders Issued	Pinnacle Duet, Uphold, Pinnacle. Polyform, Xenform, Solyx and LITE PFR Kits

CHAPTER 4

PUSHERS

"We can't afford to fall behind and be the ones chasing. Too many hands out looking for the SUI [stress urinary incontinence] business, especially in the TOT (transobturator tape) market."

—Discussion among Ethicon executives about how to handle increasing problems with the company's TVT-O sling, August 2004

"My husband began complaining that making love to me was like sleeping with a cheese grater. His penis would be cut when we had intercourse. The pain and embarrassment made me anxious, sick, and depressed."

—Mesh survivor in Australia

In a perfect world where integrity trumps greed, this would be the end of our story. As in the travesties of Vioxx and fen-phen, executives would be slammed in the press, fired, and indicted; products and drugs would be tossed from the shelves of medical offices; and future patients would be protected from becoming victims of pain and sickness from this particular device.

But this story doesn't end that way, and actions that were clearly unthinkable and unethical only escalated as doctors, sales reps, and medical device makers made millions—and even billions—off the insecurities, embarrassment, and trust of millions of women from around the world.

After the ProteGen disaster, Boston Scientific, Johnson & Johnson, and American Medical Systems returned to mesh manufacturing immediately, and other companies jumped into the frenzy as well. They tweaked their own products constantly and mimicked their competitors.

And they tested their products. Just not in live women.

Pigs, rats, sheep, and a cohort of "mongrel female dogs" in Australia were among the animals scooped up for testing at laboratories developing new vaginal mesh products for women.

And female cadavers were in demand.

But there were no serious studies on the damage those implants could cause inside a woman's pelvic area and to organs, nerves, and the muscles beyond. Boston Scientific's mea culpa—its internal promise to perform clinical trials before the next mesh implosion was also ignored—especially for any clinical trials of significant duration in living females.

There was almost no dissemination of the key negative information that Boston Scientific had found about mesh implants in the wake of its ProteGen debacle.

The stunning failure rate of 30 percent among ProteGen patients was laid at the feet of the doctors—for example, poorly trained surgeons, poorly skilled urologists operating too close to women's bladders, and their poor choice of patients.

Investors in the burgeoning female health-care industry, its member companies, and their lobbyists breathed a collective sigh of relief because the mesh implant itself was off the hook.

In fact, after the ignominious recall of ProteGen because of its dangers to women's health, many other mesh devices were actually approved for market by the FDA based on ProteGen. So here's the question: If Boston Scientific *and* the FDA knew that a device caused more harm than help, why would they approve more of the same risky products that would bring about similar outcomes?

Money. Greed. Boston Scientific knew the extent of the potential damages that certain features of their vaginal slings caused after so many patient complaints.

COMPLICATIONS AND COMPLAINTS

MDL No. 2326 filed on August 22, 2012, states: "The injuries allegedly resulting from plaintiff's use of the products at issue were not foreseeable to Boston Scientific given the state of scientific knowledge and state of the art at the time of the alleged injuries."

The "not-foreseeable" injuries that were listed in the case "include, but are not limited to, erosion, mesh contraction, infection, fistula, inflammation, scar tissue, organ perforation, dyspareunia (pain during sexual intercourse), blood loss, neuropathic and other acute and chronic nerve damage and pain, pudendal nerve damage, pelvic floor damage, and chronic pelvic pain."

Back in 1996, when Boston Scientific was preparing to launch ProteGen, the company could have tested the mesh implant and its collagen coating before putting it in thousands of vaginas. The evidence from Boston Scientific internal documents does show that the company knew a number of the most dangerous adverse effects associated with vaginal mesh, but plowed ahead anyway.

So did the other mesh makers. Within five years of ProteGen's unfortunate launch, it was followed by the In-Sling, Prolene Mesh, tension-free transvaginal taping (TVT), the TriAngle Sling, Mentor Suspend Sling, Triangle Silicone-Coated Sling, the IVS (intravaginal sling), SPARC Sling System, Sacral Colpopexy Sling, and Uretex Sup device. These were made by various manufacturers including Ethicon, American Medical Systems, Tyco Healthcare Group, and Sofradim.

Doctors had a difficult time tracking products because of the constant stream of new slings. One would be introduced to market, slightly modified to create a new and improved version, and then remarketed. While doctors should have researched the implants they were using, they were clearly chasing a moving target, and many times, the information just didn't exist. Not to mention, most doctors are so busy with their practices that they have to rely, to a large extent, on the representations and materials being provided by the medical device manufacturers, which were relayed through the companies' sales reps.

> So here's the question: If Boston Scientific *and* the FDA knew that a device caused more harm than help, why would they approve more of the same risky products that would bring about similar outcomes?

One shocking example is that when doctors searched for studies focused on the ProteGen Sling, they wouldn't be able to find any until after it was withdrawn from the market. The surgeons who implanted the ProteGen Sling from 1997 to 1999 did so without any published scientific evidence of its safety or effectiveness, but on the promises of the company's sales reps and key opinion leaders in their medical organizations.

Several researchers commented on the gap. "I am concerned that some clinicians do not appear to appreciate the true lack of evidence that accompanies most marketed devices for prolapse and incontinence. They may mistake the FDA 510(k) process of clearance for something similar to the agency's extended and complex drug approval process," wrote Dr. Anne Weber. "They may accept claims made in industry-produced white papers that are often largely promotional materials, and fail to look further into those claims."

The American Urogynecologic Society said, "Since these products are being widely used and successfully marketed with scant published data, there is very little commercial incentive to publish results."

"Without adequate information, the possibility that associated problems will not be identified until a new device has been used on hundreds or possibly thousands of women is significantly increased," concluded the AUGS statement at its 27th Annual Scientific Meeting in 2006.

In a critique of the post-ProteGen period in the mesh craze titled "The Perils of Commercially Driven Surgical Innovation," doctors in St. Louis basically asked if the urogynecology medical community had lost its mind or its ethics, or both.

"The life-cycle fiasco of the ProteGen Sling is not a unique event. The same process was repeated again within the ensuing decade," they wrote. Following the success of Ulmsten's tension-free vaginal tape (TVT) procedure, "Hordes of imitators rushed to market 'equivalent' products by creating new, potentially lucrative variations on the same theme." And the products were sold and used without remotely adequate testing, clinical trials, or reviews by regulators.

> The American Urogynecologic Society said, "Since these products are being widely used and successfully marketed with scant published data, there is very little commercial incentive to publish results."

Here's the takeaway: medical device makers weren't conducting studies, so they certainly weren't publishing them. Doctors had blind faith in the mesh they were attaching in women's vaginas. For one reason or another, thousands of doctors never even considered researching how a permanent implant would inevitably affect their patients' lives. Apparently, the average person spends more time scanning Amazon product reviews than these doctors did for a device that is intended to last the lifetime of a patient.

From roughly 1999 through 2005, the market for pelvic mesh doubled in size and kept increasing, according to a Wall Street analyst who tracked the medical device industry. Companies sold hundreds of thousands of mesh slings and then moved into full pelvic floor repair, or POP kits. "Sales went from hundreds of thousands [of dollars], to millions, to a hundred million," he said. "It was exponential."

An AARP study found that 51 percent of women ages 65 to 80 and 43 percent of women ages 50 to 64 had "an episode of incontinence in the past year and that nearly half of those who experience such leakage (48 percent) worry that their symptoms will get worse as they age." The scalability of this market and the potential for profits seemed too good to pass up.

Companies that did not have an incontinence sling in their pipeline offered "bulking" agents, silk, and biotreated filaments that absorbed liquid (i.e., urine), to prevent leakage. At least one firm spent several years on a device that used small electrical pulses to control incontinence. There were products that acted as incontinence "alarms," triggering a buzz to alert a woman that she needed to reach a restroom quickly. And, of course, there was a boom in the supply of specialty adult diapers.

But the moneymakers were the mesh implants. In the span of a few years the mesh sling for incontinence was repeatedly tweaked and put on the market as the newest innovation in incontinence repair (but not so "new" or different that the product would be required to undergo serious clinical trials).

> "Sales went from hundreds of thousands of dollars, to millions, to a hundred million," he said. "It was exponential."

There was the retropubic sling, then transurethral slings, midurethral slings, transobturator slings, and single-incision mini slings. And ironically, most of those mesh devices relied on the now-defunct ProteGen sling as their predicate product in order to pass the FDA's low standard for sale in the US.

Meanwhile, Boston Scientific, fresh off its ProteGen bust, had moved on. The company shelved its post-ProteGen "pledge" that had promised that before developing "any future sling materials, Boston

Scientific will gather clinical data to assess product performance in a broad spectrum of clinical situations."

Instead, Boston Scientific's development of future slings and pelvic meshes, as detailed in a confidential business plan in 2001, would be based on one paramount factor: "speed to market."

Anything that slowed down the sales of new products in the swelling mesh market—such as time-consuming clinical trials and continued mea culpa reviews of past mistakes—would be jettisoned.

BRING IT TO THE "BURBS"

Boston Scientific's July 2001 report, called the "Integrated Business Plan" for their developmental Advantage Transvaginal Mid-Urethral Sling System, described a veritable cornucopia of meshes that could end up on the market, as well as the menace from competition that could limit their profit takings.

"The tension-free sling marketplace will likely become crowded very soon," said Boston Scientific's report for its 13-person mesh development team. "It is estimated over 200,000 worldwide TVT procedures have been done to date. We estimate over 46,000 in the US alone since the late 1998 launch. This represents $73 Million in worldwide sales and $27 Million in US sales to date."

One of Boston Scientific's top competitors, Johnson & Johnson, would work to maintain existing customers to "ensure return on the substantial market development investments made these past 24 months." More urgently, the report said, Johnson & Johnson was expanding its gynecology base "while simultaneously aggressively expanding into urology."

That left Boston Scientific with only "a narrow window of opportunity" to "quickly" build a leading position for its Advantage sling among "urology specialists and academicians" before 2003.

The report analyzed the threat from other mesh makers such as C. R. Bard, Tyco, and American Medical Systems (AMS). Bard had been acquired by Tyco, and Tyco had a new product in the tension-free tape line, the IVS Tunneller, which might grab market share.

Pinnacle Mid-Urethral Sling System
Integrated Business Plan (IBP)
July 19, 2001

E. Initial Customer Analysis

Given current trends, competitive offerings and established segment behavior, we see the following as the driving forces in customer activity:

- As Urogynecologists continue to establish practices in the cities, the urology and gynecology female incontinence specialists respond by aggressively consolidating the patient pool. Generalists are the first to lose referrals to these emerging specialists.

- Female incontinence specialists are becoming powerful; decision- makers and profitable call-points for our TMs. While many initially sought to build their practice around a single procedure, the trend is a preference to incorporate several different approaches that are tailored for the specific patient.

- Female incontinence specialists want the least invasive sling procedure that can also minimize commonly associated sling complications. They currently attempt to reconcile a perceived trade-off between established long term durability or traditional pubo-vaginal slings with the lesser invasive, lower morbidity technologies that are not yet proven as durable.

- Reimbursement remains favorable for slings as inpatient procedures. The trend to outpatient has begun and initial APC codes are approved for all major technology options.

- There remains a clear difference in technology utilization between urologists and gynecologists. Overall, urologists support transvaginal bone anchor procedures while gynecologists are moving straight from Burch to tension-free slings.

- While we project female incontinence urologists will remain skeptical with tension-free slings throughout 2001, we are already seeing the initial trends of "experimenting" with this new approach. Bone anchors are in a more mature stage of the product life cycle. We expect tension-free slings to become a dominant threat to our anchor product line within 12-18 months.

- Speed-to-market is essential to succeed in penetrating the female urologist segment and our market modeling reflects this. It also reduces the potential number of tension-free sling competitors we would face in our first 12 months of selling tension-free slings.

Both Boston Scientific and AMS had "largely saturated" the urologist market, the 2001 report said, and would need to find more customers. American Medical Systems, now swimming in the tension-free tape pool, had launched a product named SPARC. AMS was also working on the "development of the new Staple-Tack anchor device," per the report.

Mentor, which the report called Boston Scientific's previous top rival among device makers, had shown "willingness and ability to be a significant force in the female stress urinary incontinence marketplace." Mentor did not yet have a sling procedure device to accompany their sling materials. But, the report noted, Mentor was nonetheless a "prime candidate" to enter the tension-free sling market.

Boston Scientific didn't need to worry about smaller companies entering the field anytime soon, the report said. Emerging injectable technology would only have limited impact, and drug therapy "is not promising at this time" for SUI. But there was concern that the behemoth device maker Medtronic might venture aggressively into slings, the report speculated. Why not? The overall market for slings was growing at an "impressive" 12.5 percent rate.

THE VAGINA AS BIT COIN

Basically, Boston Scientific would have to increase the number of customers, and that meant expanding its perspective of its consumer base. And the company would have to get to those new customers faster than competitors.

The growing number of urogynecologist specialists was establishing practices in "new cities," the report said. In response, urology and gynecology female incontinence specialists were "aggressively" consolidating the patient pool. "Generalists" were the first to lose referrals to the emerging specialists.

"Female incontinence specialists are becoming powerful decision-makers and profitable call-points" for Boston Scientific's marketing managers, the report said. Those female incontinence specialists "want the least invasive sling procedure that can also minimize commonly associated sling complications," although the lesser invasive technologies "are not yet proven as durable."

Although insurance and Medicare reimbursement was still covering slings as inpatient procedures, "the trend to outpatient has begun."

"We expect tension-free slings to become a dominant threat to our anchor product line within 12–18 months," the report stated.

There was only one thing to do: "Speed to market is essential" if Boston Scientific wanted to penetrate the female urologist customer base with new less-invasive tension-free slings, "and our market modeling reflects this."

Speed to market would also reduce the potential number of competitors that Boston Scientific would face "in our first 12 months of selling tension-free slings," the report concluded.

ProteGen and Boston Scientific's mistakes were, as the saying goes, tossed into the dustbin of history.

TURF WAR

Gynecare, a part of Johnson & Johnson/Ethicon, benefited from Boston Scientific's embarrassing failure with ProteGen. The company became a player in the cornucopia of mesh makers after J&J made a business agreement with the Swedish doctor Ulf Ulmsten (the "father of TVT"). J&J bought the rights to his vaginal implant procedure using plastic mesh strips and launched Gynecare's first TVT (tension-free vaginal tape) sling in Europe in 1997.

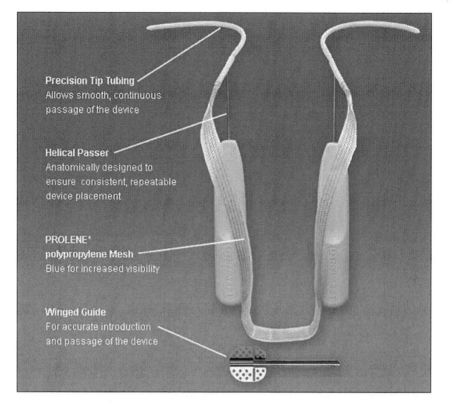

Precision Tip Tubing
Allows smooth, continuous
passage of the device

Helical Passer
Anatomically designed to
ensure consistent, repeatable
device placement

PROLENE*
polypropylene Mesh
Blue for increased visibility

Winged Guide
For accurate introduction
and passage of the device

Back in the US, the FDA cleared Gynecare's first TVT model in January 1998, just as Boston Scientific was formally recalling ProteGen. One of the iconic, perhaps comic, events in the saga of mesh is that Gynecare's TVT cited the disgraced ProteGen sling as its predicate product with the FDA, in order to pass through the US government's fast-track loophole. ProteGen's withdrawal conveniently left a brief vacuum in the nascent incontinence vaginal mesh market. Gynecare quickly filled that gap, making it temporarily the leader in the mesh race.

Johnson & Johnson has always excelled at sales ideas and strategies to build a market. Its Gynecare division was pushed to manufacture and market a second-generation TVT product and other pelvic floor repair devices to maintain a competitive advantage.

Other companies wanted a piece of the mesh craze, and Boston Scientific was planning its comeback product. Gynecare complained that competitors were "hijacking" the success of its TVT. The influx of new meshes forced Gynecare to push newer products quickly onto the market.

In 2002, Gynecare launched Project Mulberry, the development of its TVT-Obturator sling model, or TVT-O. The product used a novel "inside-out" obturator approach created by a Belgian professor; it was intended to decrease the risk of major vessel, bowel, and bladder injury from the incontinence sling's implant.

By this time, Gynecare was in a race with American Medical Systems, which was in the process of developing their own version of the obturator approach, according to a legal analysis of the project.

To reach the market first, Gynecare skipped clinical testing and instead relied on the limited studies performed in Belgium. The TVT-O was critical to Ethicon/Gynecare's moves to "expand and protect the TVT market."

In the "speed to market" mania, TVT-O was rushed into sale without clinical trials in order to capture a competitive advantage. "Project Mulberry is critical to Gynecare's success in the incontinence marketplace . . . We MUST make this project happen in a short period of time," said an email from an Ethicon/Gynecare VP of R&D to several recipients on June 24, 2003.

To meet the company goal of a nine-month launch phase, defendants decided to forgo any clinical studies of the TVT-O, even though one of Ethicon's VPs had suggested that the medical team conduct six months of clinical testing. Several outside consulting urogynecologists— termed "preceptors"—had expressed concerns about the safety of the novel "inside-out" approach in TVT-O, and the longer learning curve they believed doctors would require. In fact, the Belgian professor even expressed concern regarding the product's design.

Gynecare submitted its 510(k) application for TVT-O on schedule in November 2003. The device received approval by the FDA only 25 days later and was launched in January 2004. But American Medical Systems beat Gynecare's TVT-O to market. The two companies chased each other's tails over the next several years.

STRUGGLING TO REMOVE A
PERMANENT IMPLANT

The TVT slings and the ersatz TVTs came and went during the mesh gold rush between 1997 and 2005, keeping Wall Street satisfied with their rising sales numbers. But other kinds of numbers were rising also—the side effects of mesh slings.

And so, several doctors began developing their own techniques and honing their skills at something that mesh makers had not planned for—mesh "removal."

Dr. Dionysios Veronikis, who supported incontinence sling implants and performed many of them, remembers doing his first mesh removal when he was at Massachusetts General in the mid-1990s. By 1998, he said in interviews for this book, "You could already see which models were likely to cause problems for women."

Veronikis has practiced in St. Louis for the past 21 years. He doesn't do prolapse mesh implants. He still performs incontinence sling implants, but only uses mesh that he measures and cuts himself for the individual patient. "I use mesh in a very specific way. I don't use the manufacturers' instructions. I believe that technique for putting it in makes it worse for patients," he said. "I developed my own technique for vaginal placement. It needs to be done by skilled people in order to get the best outcomes." But he notes, using only skilled surgeons to implant mesh isn't going to help a mesh maker increase its market.

And one of the urologists who had been flown by Ethicon to Sweden to learn sling implants from the originators, Dr. Alan Garely, was also removing them by the late 1990s, he said in interviews. He briefly became involved in the development of Covidien-Tyco's IVS Tunneller. "I was in the initial group for using it. That device was really what stopped me from implanting transvaginal mesh from kits," he said in interviews. "That was the last one I ever got involved with."

The Tunneller was one of the first kits, he said, though it wasn't a POP kit. The FDA cleared it under the 510(k) loophole in 2001. The Tunneller's predicate was Ethicon's Gynecare TVT System—which used the infamous ProteGen as a predicate.

"I was putting it [the Tunneller] in and teaching other doctors at the same time," said Garely.

"I put in 12 of them. And I think I had 9 erosions . . . That's when I immediately stopped implanting. I thought, based on the technique of the procedure, I worried I was going to teach someone to kill a patient. I wasn't going to be part of that," he said. "I told the company reps about the problems I saw, and said 'No thank you, I'm done.'"

That was around 2002. The Tunneller became one of the leading examples used by medical studies reviewing side effects from mesh implants that had somehow ended up on the market and inside women during the rush of 1998–2005.

SPARC-ING PROFITS

American Medical Systems' mesh saga demonstrates how easily a company could amass wealth during the Cornucopia of Mesh period. And how easily a company could lose it.

AMS was a relatively small device maker based in Minnetonka, Minnesota, with a nice solid division selling urology implements and devices to treat male incontinence and sexual functionality. In 2000, the company went public with an IPO. In total, the first nine months of 2000 boasted net sales of nearly $77 million, a 23 percent increase over the first nine months of the previous year.

With its stable position in the male urology market, it was natural that as female incontinence slings became the market rage, AMS would join in.

During an earnings call in 2000, AMS signaled its move to market mesh. Its CEO announced the company would soon introduce a "next-generation sling procedure" for female patients suffering from stress urinary incontinence using less invasive surgery. In 2001, as Boston Scientific predicted, AMS launched the first TVT mesh sling to be inserted through the vaginal wall. It was called SPARC.

The following year, the Minneapolis *Star Tribune* said AMS stock had become "one of the top-performing medical technology companies of any size in the past 12 months." True, AMS had benefited from "the Viagra craze," the paper noted. However, its newest product line had also proved a winner: female incontinence products for women grew in the "mid–20 percent range."

The company's CEO, Doug Kohrs, said about 75 percent of the company's 2001 incontinence revenue came from products for men, but he expected that revenue from men's and women's products would be about equal by 2003. After that, he said, "Female incontinence is growing faster," and AMS was ready for it, according to the *Star-Tribune*.

During an earnings call in 2002, a reporter asked for an update from the AMS Women's Health division and in urinary incontinence.

Rival Boston Scientific had recently boasted during its third-quarter earnings conference "about a 50 percent increase in their pelvic floor business," the reporter said. Now the similar business of AMS was also skyrocketing, with 43 percent growth. The reporter asked, "Is the market really this robust?"

Oh, yes it was, CEO Kohrs responded. "I said in the past that I believe that the female incontinence market itself is growing at about a 35, 30 to 35 percent rate, just overall market growth." He added that American Medical Systems was growing faster than the market.

American Medical Systems launched its new mesh sling in that same year. In 2003, the company reported a stunning 48 percent revenue growth in its Women's Health division in the first quarter over the previous year.

That surge continued with AMS beating earnings estimates quarter after quarter for several years, and a key part of its success was its female incontinence mesh products. In 2004, it introduced the BioArc SP sling.

Although AMS had been a latecomer to the incontinence mesh slings, it jumped ahead of its competitors in the new prolapse mesh trend beginning in 2004. It launched the first vaginal mesh implants for prolapse, its POP kits Apogee and Perigee, while Ethicon and Boston Scientific were still developing their models.

The new chief executive of AMS sounded elated during the company's third-quarter earnings call in 2005. "Now let me highlight for you the depth of our revenue growth. Our women's health business reported revenues of $21 million and a growth rate of nearly 41 percent over the third quarter of 2004," he said, adding that the strong revenue growth came from the female incontinence business.

"We are clearly the market leader in the surgical treatment of stress incontinence," he said. AMS anticipated that its full-year revenue growth for female incontinence would be "12 to 14 percent on a year-over-year basis."

(AMS' other products that monetized the vagina weren't doing as well as mesh, but were still performing. The "Her Option" machine, designed to treat heavy menstrual bleeding, achieved "record revenues" in 2005. "Our business model was to place machines in physicians' offices on a per-use fee basis," the CEO said. He added, "We are seeing an increasing number of these physicians opt to purchase a 'Her Option' machine.")

Then the CEO delivered the best news: AMS' "innovative products for prolapse," Perigee and Apogee, had delivered, as anticipated, significant growth.

PFR Kit - Anterior Apical

Program Objective:

-Approval of revised "quick knock-off
Perigee with benefits" PFR Kit strategy

PIB Decisions Requested:

- Agree to new PFR kit strategy & contract
- Move into Proposal Phase
- Resource Approval for the project
- Begin immediately after resources are available

"We trained approximately 470 additional physicians this quarter on these two revolutionary products. We anticipate that we will train an additional 460 physicians before year end," said the CEO. AMS estimated that the prolapse business would add an incremental $15–$17 million to the women's health business in 2005.

The AMS Women's Health division, driven by its incontinence and prolapse slings would continue to grow and hold its market share, making it a great acquisition target for larger medical corporations. Sure enough, in 2011, Endo Pharmaceuticals paid $2.9 billion to buy American Medical Systems.

Then the mesh lawsuits started coming in and the medical device makers could no longer hide the truth.

THE MENTOR OBTAPE NIGHTMARE

Boston Scientific's 2001 "Speed to Market" report mentioned its concern with mesh options available to Mentor, a leading rival. Mentor wished to become a player in the mesh market. As Boston Scientific guessed, the California-based Mentor and its French partner company Porgès were planning their own version of a TVT product, which they would launch in the US in 2003.

That implant, the transobturator "ObTape," has been described as one of the worst device flops of the entire pelvic mesh debacle. Mentor's ObTape shows how the "speed to market" frenzy led to life-changing damages for many women.

The Mentor story is also important for understanding how multinational companies played the US FDA and the American medical market, successfully controlling the spread of negative information about their mesh products.

When Mentor moved into mesh, it looked at the competition among existing stress incontinence sling models Most pelvic meshes were a version of polypropylene woven mesh. The standard poly mesh was flexible—it was supposed to be that way in order to be fitted perfectly inside the pelvis.

What if Mentor offered doctors a "stiffer" mesh?

The company produced a nonwoven polypropylene mesh. The tape was threaded underneath the urethra, through the vagina, and then through the obturator foramen, which is near the top of patients' legs. The FDA cleared the ObTape in July 2003 as "substantially equivalent" to other predicate devices for sale in the US.

In the article "The Perils of Commercially Driven Surgical Innovation," the writers cited the Mentor ObTape as proof that, in the wake of the ProteGen implosion, "history repeats itself."

ObTape sales boomed. At the end of 2004, the year after its launch, Mentor's Women's Health Products division posted fourth-quarter revenues of $5.6 million, an increase of 89 percent over the fourth quarter of 2003. Mentor ascribed the jump in that division as "driven by sales of Mentor's ObTape device for stress incontinence." Mentor's ObTape had already been used in over 20,000 cases.

"Alas, however, the honeymoon was not to last. A cascade of complications soon followed, and the product was withdrawn from the market in 2006," according to "The Perils of Commercially Driven Surgical Innovation."

Like the events in the case of the ProteGen Sling disaster, the damage to patients from the ObTape was largely done before the complications were reported in medical journals or had been related to the urogynecology community in the US. "Once again, a defective product was cleared for sale without clinical proof of its safety and efficacy, and as a result, it entered the market, where it was pushed relentlessly by commercial interests, doing immeasurable harm to patients," the article said.

That damning article was published in 2010, after the ObTape had disappeared from the market, but before more internal Mentor documents were released, revealing astounding corporate behavior.

Mentor actually first launched its ObTape in 2002—in France—the year before its clearance in the US.

To make a "stiffer" mesh, Mentor decided on a poly mesh whose shape was solidly welded, as if pressed by an iron or waffle maker. It was not woven and did not have pores or holes. In fact, Mentor had sold an earlier version of nonwoven, welded ObTape in Europe, called UraTape. Mentor had added a patch of silicone to UraTape to enhance its smoothness. It was a novel scientific approach, which like the other meshes, was not tested first in women. UraTape was relatively quickly and quietly removed from the market in Europe after a number of complaints.

The company's scientists thought the problem with UraTape was its silicone patch. Therefore, with their next version, the ObTape, they did not add a silicone patch to the sling. Problem solved.

Nonetheless, complaints and concerns about the safety of ObTape began coming in at an alarming rate. By May 2004, according to court documents, ObTape had shown a higher rate of complications in France than other products. Furthermore, its complications seemed worse. That year, the inventor of ObTape, Dr. Emmanuel Delorme, stopped using ObTape and began using a macroporous, woven mesh product instead. But doctors in the US didn't know that the ObTape's inventor had stopped using his own product.

A study in the *Journal of Urology* in 2005 explained the scientific drawbacks of nonwoven ObTape: "The success of any synthetic sling is predicated on its satisfactory integration and incorporation, attributed to tissue in-growth of fibroblasts and macrophages between the poly-propylene filaments." In other words, the one thing worse than stan-dard polypropylene mesh with pore holes is mesh without them. The macroporous tape with large pore openings allows tissue to grow and attach itself, stabilizing the sling (at least in theory).

The nonporous ObTape was not acting like an implant, but like a marauder. And without pores, the mesh was a perfect incubator for bacteria.

ObTape's stiffness would create additional problems. "Stiff, non-woven, inelastic synthetic slings may not conform to the surround-ing tissue as well as the more elastic slings, further interfering with integration," said the study titled "Vaginal Mesh Extrusion Associated with Use of Mentor Transobturator Sling."

These problems became the focus of one of the mesh industry's top medical consultants, Dr. Michel Cosson. Cosson was talking regularly with people at Mentor about its incontinence sling, but he didn't like the bad news he was hearing about ObTape in French women.

Dr. Cosson and his colleagues were already tracking those issues of ObTape in 2004. He told French Mentor employees that the serious side effects with ObTape were caused by the melded material of the sling. Dr. Cosson made recommendations to Mentor about how to advise physicians on what to do in the event of complications—remove the mesh from the patient. But, he says, Mentor did not issue his suggested actions.

"I thought they had listened to me," Cosson said in an interview for this book. "I was very clear about what I found, what many French doctors had found with the ObTape."

In the case of unusual infection—even if it wasn't in the patient's vagina—Cosson said doctors should look at the mesh in the patient. "They would see what had happened," he said. Doctors everywhere needed to know that at the first sign of complications, the mesh had to be taken out, as much as possible, Cosson said.

That was crucial, he stated, because it would save the doctors and the women months of useless treatments for the wrong condition, while infection from the mesh continued to spread.

Cosson was becoming a bit of a nuisance for the company. Concerned about Mentor's seemingly slow response to him, he conducted a survey of his French colleagues on the side effects involving slings.

Then he published an editorial in a French medical journal about the "non-negligible" risks of infection from mesh. In a nation full of rabid soccer fans, Cosson alluded to the penalties for bad behavior on the field in the editorial's title, "Time-Out or Red Card."

After listing the reasons the transobturator tape could lead to infection, Cosson's article politely trashed the way the tape was designed to be placed. "Of greater concern is the fact that this technique seems to result in a higher rate of pelvic cellulitis [a bacterial infection involving the inner layers of the skin]," he wrote. "Probably because the transobturator tape goes through the thigh muscles, opening up potentially larger areas where infection could spread. Several cases of abscess formation have been described following the insertion of UraTape-type tapes."

Cosson was, unfortunately, prescient.

The article ended with the soccer analogy—the symbolic red card "should suggest that certain manufacturers and certain tapes should leave the playing field, either temporarily or definitively."

Mentor decided not to respond to the editorial. "It might trigger off another article from Cosson, with more solid facts, and details of the UraTape and ObTape's serious cases," read an internal company email.

By early 2005, the French health authorities and doctors became concerned that the ObTape adverse events had been significantly underreported to them, or reported late. The French health ministry then conducted a survey of mesh products on the French market and determined that ObTape had the highest complication rate.

"Complications" sounds innocuous. In fact, women in France developed terrible infections that quickly spread to other parts of their bodies, confusing doctors as to the cause. The infections didn't immediately respond to standard antibiotic treatments. Some 14 ObTape patients in France were put into hyperbaric sterile chambers, where they received anaerobic antibiotics via injection.

Two of Mentor's top French employees dealing with ObTape, and talking with Cosson, raised their concerns to superiors about the need to notify doctors about the side effects. The French employees, Dr. Catherine Ortuno and Nathalie Gremaud, were apparently perceived as overreacting to information about complications, according to internal Mentor emails.

But other Mentor/Porgès employees in France also worried. In June, a senior scientist wrote, "We have to deplore more and more the ObTape post-implantation erosion/infection problems . . . with often dramatic consequences for the patients." He continued, "We no longer count (in a way of speaking . . .) urologists who decide to stop using ObTape in favor of competitors' mesh."

In August 2005, Ortuno and Gremaud sent a report to their superiors detailing their concerns that the nonporous, heat-welded mesh was responsible for the side effects. They recommended that Mentor pull ObTape from the market in France.

The next month, the chief of Mentor's French division sent an email to several employees including Ortuno and Gremaud telling them to maintain "full radio silence" about the ObTape drama.

Dr. Ortuno was told by Mentor she needed to talk with the company's Washington, DC–based regulatory consultant. That person is a prominent US pharmaceutical and medical device lawyer who specializes in FDA issues, including approvals and recalls. The lawyer defended ObTape's safety to Ortuno, but she said that did not change her mind about the product's dangers and the injuries already linked to the tape in France, according to testimony.

On January 4, 2006, the French government's bureau overseeing medicine and medical devices asked Mentor's representatives to contact them as soon as possible. French regulators said they were very concerned about injuries to dozens of French women who had been implanted with ObTape. Ten days later, the French health ministry "demanded" a meeting with company officials about problems with the ObTape mesh sling.

At the meeting, which took place on February 1, the French government, to paraphrase *The Godfather*, made Mentor an offer that they could not refuse:

"Either Mentor-Porgès spontaneously withdraws from the market and . . . recalls all ObTape—then no additional publicity will be made on this issue," said Mentor's internal follow-up memo.

Or, French regulators told Mentor, they were prepared to publish "an official demand of product withdrawal and recall," plus a patient's follow-up report.

Mentor's memo ended: "They gave us 10 days to send them our comments and proposals."

The company responded quickly, according to attorney Katherine Cornell of the Blizzard law firm in Texas, who represented women in the US suing Mentor over its ObTape. Mentor sold off the stock in its French warehouses in other global markets. "The company could legitimately tell the government that it was no longer selling ObTape in France—well, there were no ObTape kits available there to sell," said Cornell in interviews.

There was no publicity in France about a formal withdrawal of the product from the market, and there was nothing that could reach America and "alarm the FDA and doctors there," Cornell added.

Meanwhile, Mentor was moving on to their next product in the cornucopia of mesh, Aris. And just like that, the saga of ObTape was over.

During this time, one might ask, what was happening in the US? Weren't there similar injuries?

Yes. But that wasn't well known by doctors, the public, or apparently, US regulators, said Cornell.

Doctors in the US were not formally notified when ObTape was

> Mentor sold off the stock in its French warehouses in other global markets. "The company could legitimately tell the government that it was no longer selling ObTape in France—well, there were no ObTape kits available there to sell," said Cornell in interviews.

pulled from the market in France; they continued to implant the mesh until Mentor simply stopped selling it in America later that year.

Technically, Mentor's ObTape was never withdrawn in France or the US and there were no "recalls."

Mentor successfully "kept everything under wraps," says Cornell.

However, this would not be the final time that the US would be the last to learn about serious problems with vaginal mesh occurring in foreign countries.

SUI AND POP: THE QUICK VERSION

This would be a good place to discuss the difference between stress
urinary incontinence (SUI) and pelvic organ prolapse (POP). The mesh
to treat the first condition led to more—lots more—mesh for the second condition.

SUI is when a woman laughs, coughs, or sneezes, and then leaks
urine. The sling supports the tube that urine passes through (called the
urethra) and the neck of the bladder (where the bladder connects to the
urethra) to help prevent leaks. The condition usually occurs in women
in their mid-40s or older, or after one or more childbirths.

Slings for stress urinary incontinence are commonly referred to as "tapes." The mesh is cut into a thin strip much like a piece of Scotch tape.

The two main types of slings are pubovaginal and suburethral. A pubovaginal sling has a minimally invasive surgery; there is a small vaginal incision where the sling is placed under the urethra to support the organ. A suburethral sling sits around the urethra and is actually attached to the abdominal wall. This is a more invasive procedure and requires a couple of days in the hospital following the surgery.

Mesh used for pelvic organ prolapse is somewhat different. Our organs are usually held firmly in place by connective tissue and muscles. But due to age, pregnancy, or obesity, this connective tissue in the pelvic floor area may become weaker. POP occurs when some of the vaginal walls are weakened; then the bladder, rectum, small bowel and/or uterus sag near or in the vaginal opening. Symptoms can include pain during sex, abdominal pressure, frequent constipation, leaking urine, and back pain.

Basically, there four basic stages of POP defined by how far the bladder, womb, or bowel may have drooped. If a woman is in the later—third or fourth stages—it means that her vagina is bulging centimeter by centimeter out of her vaginal opening. Most women do not suffer severe—stages 3 or 4—prolapse. But it's usually at that point that a doctor suggests some kind of surgical intervention.

It takes more than a skinny tape-like device to hold all these organs in place or push them back where they belong. This mesh device may be wider; it may have more straps to attach it to tissue and can be used to support these organs like a hammock. However, the important thing to remember is that it's all plastic mesh—that means it has the potential to erode, puncture organs, and cause chronic pain.

Depending on her age, whether the woman wants to have more children, or the severity of the prolapse, several treatments are available: having a hysterectomy, using a pessary (a removable spongelike device) to help support the organs, or surgery. There are several different types of surgeries: one, called obliterative surgery, narrows or closes off the vagina to provide support for prolapsed organs. However, there is one major downside to this procedure—sexual intercourse is no longer possible.

There are also reconstructive surgery options, some using native tissue from the patient, usually from a tendon, and others using surgical mesh. The procedures are explained by the American College of Obstetricians and Gynecologists:

- Fixation or suspension using your own tissues (also called "native tissue repair"). This is used to treat uterine or prolapse. The prolapsed part is attached with stitches to a ligament or a muscle in the pelvis.
- Colporrhaphy—Stitches are used to strengthen the vagina so that it once again supports the bladder or the rectum.
- Sacrocolpopexy—Surgical mesh is attached to the front and back walls of the vagina and then to the sacrum (tailbone). This lifts the vagina back into place.
- Sacrohysteropexy—Used to treat uterine prolapse when a woman does not want a hysterectomy. Surgical mesh is attached to the cervix and then to the sacrum, lifting the uterus back into place.
- Vaginal mesh implant surgery—Used to treat all types of prolapse. Can be used in women whose own tissues are not strong enough for native tissue repair. "Vaginally placed mesh has a significant risk of severe complications, including mesh erosion, pain, infection, and bladder or bowel injury. This type of surgery should be reserved for women in whom the benefits may justify the risks." [Good for ACOG for providing this warning!]

In 2004, the FDA cleared transvaginal mesh for POP surgeries. (The agency classified the POP mesh as Class II—moderate risk.) In the subsequent 10 years that followed, more than 40 companies began manufacturing mesh devices. By 2012, approximately 100,000 surgeries for POP were performed annually in the United States.

CHAPTER 5

DO NO F****** HARM!

> "You know, dammit, we all took an
> oath: Do no f***** harm."
>
> —Dr. Tom Margolis, 2019

There was one doctor, however, who saw firsthand the dangers of vaginal mesh here in the United States and has been voicing his concerns almost since its inception: Dr. Michael Thomas Margolis. In this story of many antiheroes, Dr. Margolis has become a beacon of hope for many women desperate for help to remove their mangled pelvic mesh.

It started back in 1998, when a young sales rep for Ethicon paid a call on Dr. Margolis. "He was a nice-looking young guy right out of college, nicely dressed, nice kid. He comes into my office and asks if we could sit down and talk about 'this new thing that we have.'"

Margolis said, "Sure."

Ethicon's rep pulled out a mesh sling, and said, "You gotta see this. It's great, and we would like you to use this."

Margolis looked at the mesh. Ethicon was preparing to launch it as the Gynecare TVT retropubic sling; the corporation had a lot of money and its future in the mesh market riding on the product.

"I basically told the kid to get out of my office. He was doing his pitch, and said, 'Won't you listen to me first?'"

Margolis said, "You just insulted me."

The kid was looking around. "How did I insult you?"

"You just called me a stupid SoB."

He exclaimed, "I didn't call you a stupid SoB!"

"Yeah you did." Margolis told him, "You came to me, and you showed me a device that is clearly a f****** disaster."

The kid was really nervous now, and says, "What do you mean?"

Margolis said, "First of all, this device is going to cause direct trauma to all sorts of organs because the TVT trocars [implant tools] are so big, they are going to have all kinds of injuries to adjacent organs. The other thing that is a grave concern is that you want me to implant a synthetic nonabsorbable permanent material through a contaminated field into a woman's pelvic area. You can't make that sterile. You're going to get infections galore. This mesh is going to get infected and it's going to be a disaster.

"The patients are going to have problems. The doctors are going to have problems. Your company will have to deal with those problems. Are you ready for them?"

The rep left. Says Margolis, "I didn't mean to scare him."

MESH MILLS

Over a series of interviews, Dr. Margolis talked about his long and frustrating relationship with vaginal mesh, the doctors who defend it, and the many ways mesh injuries keep shocking him.

Ethicon moved forward, and as the makers and the stock market predicted, its mesh sling was an instant hit with the urogynecological community. Margolis recalls, "There were doctors in San Jose who were bragging to all their colleagues, 'I'm making a lot of money. It's a quick surgery, it's an easy surgery, requires no skill or very little skill. It's done as an outpatient. I'm making good money off this.'

"And yes, there were 'mesh mills,'" said Margolis.

"I know a lot of doctors who jumped on the mesh bandwagon. But in a short period of time they jumped right back off, when they had to explain to women, to their faces, why they were in horrible pain, bleeding—all that."

Margolis says he wasn't the only surgeon who had reservations. One of the concerns was there was no clinical data on its safety. "They hadn't tried this [mesh] in women!" says Margolis.

"It sold like hotcakes at first, then all the complications occurred. Some doctors started to see complications in their own patients—and they were experienced surgeons. They got out of it," Margolis recalls.

"Within a couple months of that guy, the sales rep, coming to my office, I got the first phone call from another doctor I knew, about a patient who had complications with it," said Margolis. "The doctor asked me, 'Tom, do you have any ideas?'

"It was the Gynecare TVT retropubic—the same model that the sales rep was pushing," Margolis said. "So the first mesh implant I took out was in 1998. Within about four months of launch of the device I was removing it."

Hold for a moment: the time period was 1998–99. Tom Margolis was starting to do mesh removals. But at the very same time, mesh makers like J&J/Ethicon, American Medical Systems, C. R. Bard, and Boston Scientific were going full tilt with new mesh creations, launching updated versions of their first generation of slings (and developing larger prolapse mesh kits back in their labs).

Margolis wasn't the only doctor trying "explants" that early in the sling craze. Across the country, Drs. Dionysios Veronikis, Alan Garely, and Shlomo Raz—surgeons who initially had high hopes for incontinence implants—were all finding their way "using trial and error," through complex "removal" procedures that medical devices makers had never planned for.

This incongruity—the initiation of mesh removal operations while mesh sling sales were skyrocketing—was the signal that doctors in the elite surgical and urogyn community missed. Mesh makers like Ethicon were funding study after study to support the safety and efficacy of mesh, but researchers should have publishing articles in medical journals about the severity of the complications and ways to address them.

And mesh complications, if mentioned at all, were discussed in sterile terms—"bothersome" side effects, "some" discomfort, increased incontinence, "occasional" blood in the urine, and dyspareunia, or "discomfort" during intercourse.

Nobody was writing about women literally screaming in pain, doubled over, with pieces of blue plastic threads hanging out of their vaginas, bloody adult diapers, and the sounds of their husbands' yelps when a sharp edge of eroded mesh nipped their penises.

What else could go wrong?

Margolis admits that even he was not prepared for the mesh complications that began piling up. "My initial concern was these were going to cause infections. I had no idea of the plethora of other complications the mesh was going to be associated with."

For example, shrinkage. "I didn't know it would shrink like that."

"I had *no* idea about the chronic scarring, the nerve entrapment, delayed obstruction, dyspareunia, deformation of vaginal canal, scarring of vagina, damage to the urethra, and rectum.

"I had no foggy idea. That's what made me more and more frustrated as the years went by. I was seeing more and more bizarre side effects in mesh implant patients.

"I didn't know about erosions. Or that the mesh could and would 'migrate.'"

When the mesh migrates around the spine, it causes nerve entrapment, Margolis explained. "I have women who are in wheelchairs or who can barely walk. The nerves that move legs or flex feet have become wrapped up in mesh that has no business around the spine.

"Did I think: 'Oh, mesh might cause ambulatory problems?' Nope, did not see that coming."

There were more surprises in store for Margolis. "I knew the mesh was going to obstruct urethras. But I thought it was going to cause urethra obstruction because doctors would put it in too tight. Not that it would migrate and cut the urethra or the bladder."

One particularly interesting complication is called "chronic foreign body giant cell reaction."

"I had never heard of that. I had to look it up," says Margolis. "Pathologists kept writing it in patient medical reports. So I called a pathologist to ask, 'Sorry to sound stupid, but what the hell is a chronic foreign body giant cell reaction?'"

Margolis was told it is histologic evidence that the immune system of the patient is attacking this mesh—in perpetuity. "But since the immune system can't get rid of the mesh, it keeps sending out these giant cells to kill it—like sending out the Terminator. But the giant cells can't destroy the mesh completely."

Margolis says there's no proof linking mesh to autoimmune disease. However, many women with mesh implants have chronic inflammatory issues that manifest themselves in unusual conditions, such as lupus. "But there's no data showing mesh causes that disease in these women," he says.

"I wasn't expecting these hideous complications."

Of the over 600 explants he has performed, he says he learned explanting by trial and error "because there is no instruction book on how to take this crap out.

"The companies planned this as a 'one-way street surgery.' Because the companies never anticipated the need to remove the mesh, I learned how to take it out by viewing all these complications, by scratching my head and going into the operating room.

"I learned by blood, sweat, and tears, employing my understanding of anatomy, developing an understanding of how mesh interacts with the body, and going in there and slugging it out."

Margolis employed all the surgical techniques he already knew, studied all the different sling and POP mesh devices, watched implant videos, reviewed the IFUs (instructions for use), which he said, "sometimes made me furious. Did they have any idea what they were doing?"

"To this day, the IFUs don't include instructions for how to remove mesh. Now they say that it might need to be removed, but they still give no guidance on how."

Margolis admits he has become a little pessimistic. Perhaps more than a little.

"I end up with these other doctors' patients. I'm fixing somebody's disaster every day. They're mangling women. And you know, dammit, we all took a f****** oath: 'Do no f****** harm!'

"I'm really frustrated," said Margolis.

"When you hear doctors say, 'I put in slings all my life and they're never a problem,' you might want to ask them, 'Have you seen your patients later on?' You know, studies show that 50 percent of the women with sling complications don't go back to the implant doctor," he notes.

Doctors are loathe to concede major problems with vaginal mesh. Margolis said, "I have been known to say that in some doctors the letters 'MD' stands for 'malignant denial.'

"The overwhelming majority of docs that I know, even bad ones, are trying to help. When there's a bad outcome, it's hard to look a patient in the eye and say, 'I tried to help you out, but I really screwed you up instead.'"

In the last several years, Dr. Margolis, who still volunteers in clinics in developing countries, has become a key expert witness for plaintiffs suing mesh companies. The money he makes—which corporate defense attorneys have calculated to the dime and love to flag to jurors—allows him to do pro bono medical care, including for many of the mesh victims who come to his practice in the San Francisco Bay Area.

But the part-time role as a witness against mesh makers—particularly Johnson & Johnson—hasn't endeared him to the medical associations (and lobbying groups) for urogynecological surgeons and ob-gyns such as the American Urogynecologic Society and the American College of Obstetricians and Gynecologists.

Conveniently, Margolis feels the same way about them.

"AUGS and ACOG are homes to a lot of well-paid KOLs—key opinion leaders for corporations like mesh makers, who fund the medical groups." In fact, corporations do more than that. "Companies are actual members of AUGS," says Margolis.

"Let's be real frank. These groups, and those KOLs and consultants receive millions of dollars from companies. When I saw that these professional associations were continuing to promote this mesh material and continuing to deny vehemently that there were any problems, it made me very disappointed and angry.

"I wrote to AUGS and asked them to disclose the financial ties, to come forward with their own personal conflicts of interest. They basically flipped me off. How did that make me feel? Let's say I was deeply disappointed in my colleagues.

"AUGS is the mouthpiece of industry," Margolis says. "AUGS is paid by industry, and when an AUGS official is being deposed in the national mesh litigation, the MDL, they are represented by industry-paid lawyers.

"AUGS and its officials and many members have a significant conflict of interest—AUGS gets paid a lot by industry, and industry expects AUGS to defend their product. And unlike me, industry is never disappointed."

In one noted surgeon's deposition, he said that one of AUGS' position papers supporting vaginal mesh use was written in part to defend doctors against lawsuits, Margolis said, citing the deposition witness.

"AUGS is and always has been a special interest group." But he's been a member in good standing for 20 years and "they absolutely hate that I am," says Margolis.

> "AUGS and its officials and many members have a significant conflict of interest—AUGS gets paid a lot by industry, and industry expects AUGS to defend their product. And unlike me, industry is never disappointed."

When he began testifying against mesh makers and nudging AUGS about vaginal mesh damages, the organization—whose members include corporations—started "looking for reasons to boot me," Margolis says.

"I was shown an email chain with a top AUGS member writing to AUGS leadership, asking 'Has he paid his dues?'"

"You bet I have," confirms Margolis.

He thinks it's unbelievable that AUGS and ACOG are still supporting mesh. AUGS, in particular, says the problems with vaginal mesh are due to poor surgical techniques and mistakes during implantation.

Asked about that, Margolis replies with a few words that can't be printed.

Then he says, "Remember the mesh study at Stanford with its 16 percent erosion rate? They had to stop the study. Was that poor surgical technique? Those were some of the best surgeons."

"Mesh is a defective material even when implanted properly. Mesh shrinkage is well established in Ethicon's own internal documents," Margolis notes.

And if mesh itself is not the problem, then "why are the companies that still make implants going to a lighter-weight mesh? Isn't that recognition that the mesh itself is problematic?"

He states, "Look what mesh has done to these women. And you know, a number of them cannot be fixed. I have to tell those women: 'I'm sorry. I have nothing else for you. I'm sad I don't have anything else. I'm sorry I can't make you any better. I'm sorry.' What else do I say?

"Let me put it bluntly. It's sad, truthful, and hard. Sometimes medicine loses. Sometimes pathology wins."

And don't forget this started for Margolis way back in 1998. He shared his patients' experiences with colleagues, AUGS, and ACOG, and no one would listen. Just imagine how many women would have been spared if they had.

Attention Dr. Nager and Board of Directors
From: Michael Margolis
To: American Urogynecologists

Charles W. Nager, MD
President, Board of Directors
American Urogynecologic Society

2/11/14

Dear Dr. Nager,

The American Urogynecologic Society Board of Directors (AUGS BOD) has authorized and published position statements on the use of transvaginal polypropylene mesh for stress urinary incontinence and pelvic organ prolapse (Mesh/Sling). The AUGS BOD has also authorized AUGS representatives to lobby the food and drug Administration, representatives of the United States Congress and the California Medical Society in support of mesh/sling. UGS?BOD has taken a consistently pro- mesh/sling position often citing limited, select and questionably objective published data that overinflated mesh/sling position often citing limited, select and questionably objective published data that overinflated mesh/sling success rates while ignoring the huge body of evidence concerning serious, frequent, permanent and irreversible complications in women as a result of mesh/sling complications.

Not only has the AUGS BOD supported mesh/sling without restraint, profoundly minimized mesh/sling complications and misrepresented the sucess rate but the AUGS BOD and its representatives have failed to disclose significant conflicts of interest throughout this process. AUGS BOD has not acknowledged in its pro mesh/sling statements. Furthermore, at least 6 of the 13 current AUGS BOD have personal conflicts of interest with industry thus further raising serious ethical concerns.

AUGS BOD has also consistently misrepresented and exaggerated support for mesh/sling by suggesting to the lay community that AUGS BOD speaks on behalf of all AUGS members, though it does not.

I formally and respectfully request that the AUGS BOD take immediate steps to correct these issues including:

1. Immediately republish all AUGS publications in support of mesh/sling with the proper disclaimer that AUGS and its BOD have significant financial conflicts of interest.

2. Republican AUGS position statements clarifying that the AUGS BOD does not speak for all AUGS members.
3. Publish new position statements that elaborate on the nprdinaltcy high complications rate of mesh/sling.
4. Publish new position statements clarifying that the claimed success rates of mesh/sling are lower than previously reported.
5. Appoint any AUGS members to the BOD who holds opposing views on mesh/sling.

The overinflated claims of high mesh/sling success rates the underreporting of mesh/sling complication rates have been a huge disservice to women. It would be tragic to find that industry support to individuals and/or organization has contributed to this serious problem.

Respectfully submitted,

Michael T Margolis, MD, FACS, FACOG
Assistant Clinical Professor
Department of Ob/Gyn, UCLA

Responding to your letter   Tue, Feb 11, 2014 at 10: 55 PM

From: Nager, Charles

To: mtom.margolis@yahoo.com

CC: Zinnert, Michelle

Dear Dr. Margolis,

I acknowledge the receipt of your email letter to me.
A survey of AUGS members after the 2011 FDA safety communication found that 99% of our members use synthetic mesh slings. (Clemons et al FPMRS, 2013). Members of the AUGS BOD are elected by AUGS members and attempt to represent AUGS members. We agree with the FDA's statement that "The Safety and effectiveness of multi-incision slings is well-established in clinical trials that followed patients for up to one-year." The Polypropylene mesh MUS is the worldwide standard of care for surgical treatment of SUI and we stand by that statement and all the other factual statements in the position statement. We accept that our stated support for the best procedure ever developed to help women with stress urinary incontinence stated that we represent everyone's viewpoint. We will not be abiding by the requests in your letter.

Sincerely yours,

Charlie Nager

KARINA'S STORY

When ob-gyns and urogynecologists are asked about the mesh implant debacle, many of them fall back on familiar talking points: "Look at all the women who do not have problems. Have you talked with the women who had success with their mesh?"

Karina was one of those women. However, Karina's story today is a warning that even if you have no symptoms of mesh erosion or migration, you may already be damaged.

Karina and her husband, Frank, who live in California with their three children, aren't sedentary suburbanites.

"I jumped on trampolines with my kids, I love to play basketball, and always, tennis," says Karina. "We're all active."

After three vaginal births, Karina was only in her early 40s when she began having stress incontinence. "I'd lunge for the net, or jump for the ball, and I'd leak." And as a businesswoman, she didn't want to risk embarrassment during a presentation or a meeting at the office.

She'd heard about incontinence slings that could "change your life."

In November 2011, after checking out several urologists in the Bay Area, Karina received a MiniArc, made by American Medical Systems. The MiniArc is one of the single-incision mini-slings that mesh makers had been promoting as quicker and easier to implant, with fewer risks than some of the larger, older hammock slings.

In July 2011, the FDA had issued a new warning, stating that serious side effects from vaginal mesh implants like prolapse kits were "NOT rare." The agency held a two-day advisory committee meeting on mesh problems that September. But Karina didn't know that, and her urologist did not mention the FDA's worrisome warning, she says. The sling implant was a success.

"She loved the results," says Frank.

"It was the BEST THING EVER!" Karina says. "I was so happy."

She could play tennis several times a week, and play basketball; the sudden movements didn't affect her, because she had stopped leaking. "It really was the best thing I'd ever done," she says.

Karina was so excited that she told her friends, and a couple of them also had MiniArcs implanted.

Frank is a partner in a wealth management firm. He likes to find unusual opportunities to help his clients diversify their investments.

By 2016, he had noticed the number of TV ads by lawyers recruiting claimants for vaginal mesh lawsuits. "We were always looking for potential investments outside of the public domain. TVM hit a note with me; it could be good for clients," he says.

Frank analyzed some of the venture capitalists lending to law firms that were participating in the burgeoning national vaginal mesh litigation. Law firms involved in the multidistrict federal case, the MDL, would likely receive lucrative settlements, but needed large-scale loans to carry them while they awaited the outcomes and distribution of awards and fees.

Frank talked with some of the groups that had pending legal settlements. As he researched more, he began reading details about some of the extensive injuries caused by mesh implants in women.

"And suddenly it occurred to me," he says, "was that what Karina had?" Frank called his wife, who confirmed she had mesh.

Karina hadn't experienced many problems herself. But two of her friends who got MiniArcs were having serious issues. One was getting interstitial cystitis and bladder infections, and was experiencing pain during intercourse.

"I felt guilty because I had convinced them to have the surgery," says Karina. And she was worried that she could be at risk herself for similar injuries.

A friend recommended that she visit Dr. Tom Margolis, a

urological surgeon in the Bay Area who by then was renowned as a leading "mesh removal" specialist. After an examination, Margolis said he'd found evidence of some erosion and possible damage to Karina's urethra. He told her that eroding mesh often entwines itself in the vaginal walls. Karina might not need surgery immediately, but it was inevitable.

Karina went back home, talked with Frank, and they made an appointment to meet with Margolis together a few months later, in 2017.

"Margolis was not pushing to operate," said Frank. "But he was pretty clear that the degeneration of the mesh had begun, and the question for us was not 'if' but 'when.'"

Both Karina and Frank heard about mesh implant patients who, for various reasons including financial, hadn't undergone a removal procedure early on. Now it was too late for their injuries to be repaired, and the damage was permanent.

Karina says she and Frank reviewed their finances. "We had our own insurance. By the time we saw Dr. Margolis, we'd met the pretty high deductible for our policy."

"I really didn't want to lose that sling, I told Dr. Margolis," says Karina. "I loved the freedom I had with it, all the sports I could play, the things I could do without leaking." Margolis said he would perform a standard Burch procedure during the mesh removal surgery to replace the sling and mitigate future incontinence. "The surgery would be straightforward," says Karina.

But it wasn't. "The operation took longer than we expected, several hours. Dr. Margolis couldn't get out all the mesh—you know his line about getting rebar out of concrete," says Frank. Margolis removed mesh parts that could cut into Karina's nerves and repaired her urethra.

"He found a hole in my urethra that was already the size of a penny, and I hadn't had symptoms yet. He showed me the pictures. I would have had bacteria getting carried throughout my body," says Karina.

She stayed in the hospital several more days and had a catheter in for a week. "It was a tough healing process," says Karina.

"But Dr. Margolis said even his gynecological exam didn't show how large the hole was" from the mesh that bore into her urethra. It could have caused more severe problems or disability in another six to twelve months. "He couldn't tell until he opened up my pelvis," Karina says. "Imagine if I had waited!"

Karina later visited her regular gynecologist and told her about the mesh removal with Dr. Margolis. "She told me, 'I put in bladder slings all the time.' I was shocked that people are still doing this," says Karina.

"The information about the damages from mesh, and how you can have serious damage occurring even before you have symptoms—that's not getting to doctors or patients," says Karina. "That's the scariest part—that they still don't know."

CHAPTER 6

VA-CHING!

"Surgery is the cha-ching thing."

—Ethicon marketing line in "The Growth-Driven Physician"

In summer 2005, Johnson & Johnson pulled together a group of men and women to expand the sales force of its subsidiary Ethicon. The female incontinence market was exploding, according to Wall Street projections, and J&J saw the future in vaginas. The sound of cash piling up in bank accounts was able to drown outpatient complaints and the voices of concerned physicians like Dr. Margolis.

Women were already spending millions of dollars each year on incontinence products, including absorbent pads. Pharmaceutical companies were polishing new TV commercials targeting women, listening to focus groups, and carefully substituting softer words like "overactive bladder" for "incontinence."

Johnson & Johnson, best known to the average American consumer for Band-Aids, baby shampoo, and Tylenol, was rapidly expanding its empire. It had invested millions in its subsidiary Ethicon and its women's health and urology division. Core products for women's health care included devices for minimally invasive surgeries such as a laparoscopic supracervical hysterectomy (LSH) and the morcellator, a device that cut away fibroids in the uterus. The new plastic pelvic mesh implants were critical to Ethicon's growth.

But the company had to move fast (sound familiar?).

Competitors such as American Medical Systems and Boston Scientific had been selling mesh implants in the form of incontinence slings since the late 1990s. AMS, in particular, had cornered much of that area by marketing their products to urologists, urogynecologists, and pelvic reconstruction experts who were doctors with the training and the experience to adopt a new surgical skill. Additionally, AMS created loyal customers, which was bad news for J&J and Boston Scientific because, as marketing experts knew, surgeons—even more than regular doctors—are loathe to change their habits.

Furthermore, AMS was ahead in the race to develop a new category of mesh product. It was an actual kit for implanting pelvic mesh to support women's organs in the pelvic floor, repairing the prolapse that caused much of the female incontinence. There was one kit for the anterior and one for the posterior—Apogee and Perigee.

Looking at American Medical System's progress, Boston Scientific and Ethicon/J&J faced a difficult climb. The urogynecologists and pelvic reconstruction surgeons had been largely co-opted by AMS. However, those specialists represented only about 10 percent of the total physician community handling women's ob-gyn issues.

J&J and Boston Scientific had to come up with a way to expand their doctor market.

The answer was obvious: Why fight over the 10 percent of the medical community that's already made its brand choice? Instead, they decided to go after the other 90 percent—the ob-gyns.

Ob-gyns are often called primary care doctors for women, or less kindly, "baby catchers." But there was another label for those physicians that salespeople and even some corporate suits casually tossed around: the "low-hanging fruit."

Johnson & Johnson had begun thinking about revising their perspective of the doctor market as early as 2001. In one TVT sales plan, which included Ethicon/Gynecare's six-year sales projections, the market strategy focused on shifting the mesh procedures from urologists to gynecologists.

"This transfer among the provider of treatment would play to Gynecare's strengths, the gynecologist, while shifting away from the competition's strength, the urologist," the plan said, indicating the ongoing concern at J&J that AMS had captured the loyalty of the urologists and pelvic surgeons.

> Basically, the mesh makers' plan was simply to target underqualified doctors and thereby radically expand the market for mesh implants. And they succeeded.

Boston Scientific had a similar idea. In 2006, a Boston Scientific internal marketing document laid out their target audience for mesh implants. It showed a pyramid with a small triangle at the top labeled "SUI Thought Leaders & Hospital Screamers." The next section down was the "Thought Leader Followers." At the bottom, the largest part of the pyramid of doctors was labeled "low-hanging fruit."

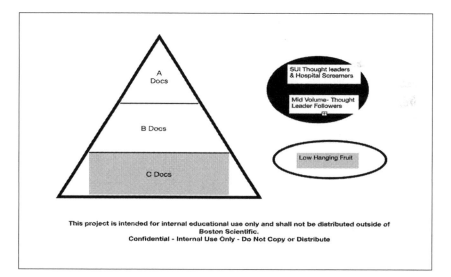

Basically, the mesh makers' plan was simply to target underqualified doctors and thereby radically expand the market for mesh implants. And they succeeded.

TRUE THAT

Being a doctor of the female anatomy is not for the faint of heart. The pelvic area starting at the vagina is a small, dark place, surrounded by major organs and blood vessels. The reproductive organs are toward the front; at the back are the bladder and the urethra, which control urination, packed tightly behind the vaginal wall. The slip of a scalpel or sharp instrument like a trocar, and you can maim a woman for life.

Ob-gyns spend four years in medical school like most MDs, then usually three more as residents, then take extra courses to pass their board certification. Urogynecologists complete all that, and then spend an additional year learning the complex surgery of the pelvic area, like urological operations and rectocele and pelvic reconstruction.

The new salespeople hired for Ethicon around 2005 were going to take a roughly six-month-long training course at the end of which they would be prepared to recruit gynecological doctors to the world of vaginal mesh. Then they would help those doctors learn to surgically implant permanent plastic mesh products in the middle of women's pelvises.

Many of Ethicon's new sales recruits at that time were relatively recent college graduates; some had little sales experience and few had any background in science, medicine, or medical products. One class even included a former baseball player and a contractor who renovated houses.

Participants were sent to J&J's campus near its headquarters in New Jersey. Early in the course, the new sales reps were taught Latin and Greek anatomical terminology.

"We learned Latin terms like medial, lateral, distal, all those kind of words that they use in surgery," said one former Ethicon sales rep in a series of interviews. "Then they began to teach us the anatomy of the vesicovaginal, which is the space between the vagina and the bladder. And about the rectal-vagina, which is the space between the rectum and the vagina," he said. "Once we got past the medical terminology, we went into the actual anatomy of a woman."

The crash course in the female body focused on the pelvic area that shelters reproductive organs, which sits very close to organs controlling urination and the bowel.

They were taught about the reigning standard procedure for female SUI, the Burch surgery, and were given well-analyzed talking points to drop in conversation when discussing the drawbacks of Burch. "We were told to tell our doctors, if their patient was past menopause or older, the Burch procedure wouldn't work, because at that age, the female patient's vaginal tissue wouldn't be strong enough."

The baby boomers' female population was now middle-aged and menopausal and replete with women who had born children. It was a large, ready-made customer base for incontinence and prolapse products. Mesh City.

"Then we got into product and competition." Reps-to-be memorized many ways to describe the joy of mesh, the substitution of plastic for natural tissue. "We were told it was a polypropylene mesh; that it had been used in Europe, Australia, and other places; and women had success. We were told it was FDA approved."

Well, not exactly. "We were told there were studies," said one ex–sales rep. But later, he said, he learned there wasn't clinical data on the vaginal mesh products. The pelvic mesh had only been "cleared" by the FDA, thanks to the 510(k) loophole in which companies could avoid testing, if a part—just about any part—of their new product had been already "approved" by the FDA in a different product, using clinical data. The standard for "clearance" was not "safety and efficacy." It was "substantial equivalence." Again, hernia mesh made from plastic had been approved by the FDA in 1985, and these new vaginal implants were also made out of plastic mesh. Good enough, right?

At the end of class sessions in New Jersey, Ethicon's student groups hit the road. "They sent us out in the fields for a couple of weeks across the country, with top surgeons and J&J's hired guns [consultants]," said an ex–sales rep. "We would actually view the surgery and learn how we could walk a physician step-by-step through this process."

Then came hands-on training with "preceptors," who were the elite private surgeons working with Ethicon. "I did an implant on a cadaver," said the ex-rep. It was not as easy as their marketing materials suggested, but that was not to be mentioned. He also said it was clear that the size—the height and weight—of the female patient would affect the complexity of the implant, another factor that wasn't highly publicized.

With some other students, this sales rep had questions about the basic tenets of the surgery. First, trying to raise the bladder and urethra from underneath seemed counterintuitive, and like trying to flout the laws of gravity. "Everyone knows it's easier to get to the pelvis from above than from below, up through the vagina . . . It's better to lift something from above than push it up from below," said the ex-rep.

Then there was the problem of visibility. In the Burch method, going into the pelvic area via an abdominal opening, surgeons could see more of their working area. But going in through the vagina was like "working blind."

Those drawbacks, however, were not going to stop the deluge of mesh products being introduced to physicians, patients, and industry investors. Mesh makers were not going to be derailed by technical questions regarding whether the mesh surgery procedures would work.

Now it was time for the trained mesh sales reps to pick "the low-hanging fruit," otherwise known as ob-gyns.

THE NEW "GOLD STANDARD"

There are about 38,000 practicing doctors in the American College of Obstetricians and Gynecologists (ACOG), a medical association which relies on funding from the medical device makers. There are guidelines regarding their standards of care for patients. And, as a general standard, they did not conduct surgery for incontinence or pelvic floor prolapse.

How would companies like J&J get them on board the Mesh Express?

To first influence these physicians, mesh makers set out to revise the paradigm. They had to change gynecologists' view of "the gold standard" for female incontinence treatment, according to numerous documents, former mesh implant surgeons, and ex–sales reps.

"It was our major talking point," said the ex-rep. "We had to change their mind-set."

We discussed the old gold standard, the Burch procedure that was practiced before Ulf Ulmsten decided to put mesh into the vagina. As a reminder, the Burch procedure took between 45 minutes to an hour and required anesthesia, then patients stayed one or more nights in the hospital. It used "native" or natural tissue from the patient to create support when rearranging the urethra and bladder positions to limit leaks. The tissue sometimes came from the patient's abdominal wall or a tendon in the patient's legs. The risks included excessive bleeding and nicks to the urethra. Sometimes incontinence returned after a few years and the surgery would need to be redone. Burch was not a procedure that patients (or doctors) easily embraced, like laser vision surgery or a tummy tuck.

From the companies' perspectives, the Burch method had another major flaw: Burch did not require the use of a shiny new medical device with very low manufacturing costs and high-profit margins. For J&J and Boston Scientific, Burch was essentially useless as a moneymaker.

Reps told ob-gyns during their visits that J&J subsidiaries, Ethicon and Gynecare, had created a whole division, Women's Health & Urology, where the new "gold standard" was driving innovation. That new gold standard would be their crown jewel: vaginal mesh.

The mesh companies also needed to convince the ob-gyn community that it was time to expand their portfolio of services to patients and stop giving away lucrative opportunities to other medical specialists. Since the launch of vaginal mesh implants in the late 1990s, ob-gyns had been referring patients with incontinence to other doctors such as urogynecologists and pelvic surgeons for the vaginal mesh "sling."

Privately, ob-gyns complained about having to sit out the new wave of incontinence treatments and watch the elite of the gynecological community waltz off with their patients and a rushing stream of revenue. That was the opening for companies like J&J and Boston Scientific. "We roped them in," said the ex–sales rep. "We played to . . . their inferiority complex."

That's how thousands of physicians with minimal or no pelvic surgery experience became mesh implant doctors for hundreds of thousands of American women.

One of the sales rep's "messages" to ob-gyns about implants played down the gap in surgical experience with urogynecologists. The reps said, "Doctor, this is a mesh, and these are handles, instruments that were made only for the hands of an ob-gyn. This mesh is made especially for your specialty."

That got the attention of the doctors, said the ex–sales rep.

In addition, "We had, like, scripts," designed to highlight the financial benefits of mesh implants. For example, "See that Lamborghini in the parking lot? That could be *your* Lamborghini, Doctor."

Sales reps said that when they made their pitch to ob-gyns, they told them the Lamborghinis or other luxury cars in medical center parking lots probably belonged to urogynecologists and pelvic surgeons, physicians with surgery privileges who charged upscale fees. "Why do you keep referring your incontinence and prolapse patients to pelvic surgeons, and sending women to other doctors, when you could be fixing those incontinence problems yourself?" the sales reps asked the doctors.

If the ob-gyn doctors learned to implant incontinence slings, or better yet, adopted the new mesh prolapse kits that were appearing on the market, they could just sit back and watch their income skyrocket. "You can implant the mesh in the time it takes to order a Domino's pizza" went the sales reps' script, boasting that this surgery could be performed in 30 minutes or less. "You can do three or four of these implants in a morning and still be on the golf course by noon." That would be roughly $10,000 in revenues, according to internal marketing documents.

SURGERY IS THE CHA-CHING THING (WHETHER YOU'RE TRAINED OR NOT . . .)

The lure of money is universal, and Ethicon had already been recruiting physicians in other countries to try out their new products before presenting them to the FDA. Sales reps with Ethicon had been working on scripts for videos or other presentations to make to gynecological doctors, according to internal J&J documents.

One such script was aimed at "the Practice-Driven Physician"— later shown as "the Growth-Driven Physician." It specified the props to include:

- Photo of an expensive car
- Photo of European ski trip
- Boating magazine
- Shirt and tie with lab coat
- (sign on back reads: "Surgery is the Cha-ching thing")

Apparently, company marketing reps hoped that a doctor's lab coat labeled with "Surgery is the Cha-ching thing" would evoke the sweet sound of a cash register.

The first script began with a physician at his desk taking a call from a colleague.

"Just got back from a week at Saint Moritz—fabulous ski conditions."

"Yeah, just picked up the Lamborghini on Friday—an amazing machine."

"And I'm finally going to invest in that sailboat this summer so we can cruise to the Caribbean."

The doctor adds that he now has a more efficient work schedule, which is enabling him to take vacations and enjoy life.

The next proposed script is the doctor getting a call from an operating room nurse. "There's an opportunity to add one more Gynecare TVT to the surgical schedule tomorrow."

"Sure. You know I can do a TVT-O in eight minutes. That makes four TVTs and an LSH before lunch."

The doctor says he's going to a health fair to talk to 50 women about pelvic conditions and treatments.

"The last two community outreach programs brought me a dozen new patients, so be prepared for a heavy surgical schedule in the next few months."

A third scene involved a call between the doctor and the rep for Ethicon's Women's Health & Urology. The doctor says he might be interested in the newest prolapse kit called Prosima.

"How's the reimbursement for that procedure? Good, good. You know I use your products because I can do more procedures in less time with better reimbursement." The doctor continues, "I can only do the training over the weekend, though. I'll be in the OR for five procedures Friday morning and have a full office schedule in the afternoon."

After the "training," doctors got a certificate of course completion from "Johnson & Johnson University" as sales reps and others in the medical device industry referred to J&J's product training system.

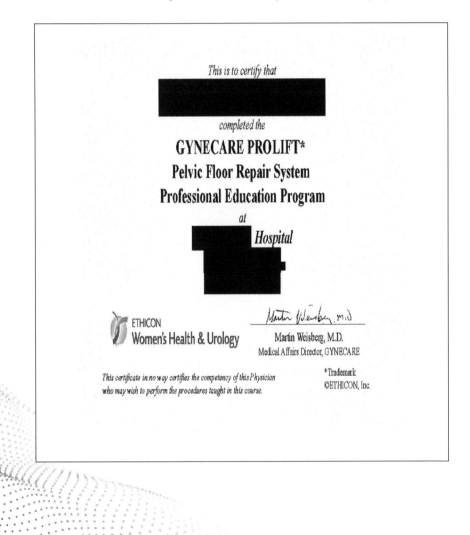

LOW-HANGING FRUIT

The weekend. Yes, two-day weekends were about long enough for busy ob-gyn doctors to learn the basics of vaginal mesh implants at one of J&J's centers. The physicians would be put up in hotels in or near popular tourist cities such as New Orleans and New York, and then they got to work.

> "We'd go out to dinner the night before training and discuss the advantages of using the mesh," explained the sales rep. "In the morning, the key opinion leader would take us into surgery, and he would have three or four patients lined up. We'd watch the doctor show them how to do it; they could scrub in and they could also touch the patient, and things like that. Made them feel comfortable." Before the sales reps left, they told the physicians that they had to agree to "stack" five patients for surgery. Repetition was the key to success, according to sales reps.

"We would fly them to Miami, wherever. We had a Johnson & Johnson University online, so we could look and see where the key doctors were" and then register an ob-gyn in a small, select group for the weekend course.

The key opinion leader—a well-known gynecological doctor, probably a prominent member of ACOG, would receive an honorarium for leading the weekend session. "We'd go out to dinner the night before training and discuss the advantages of using the mesh," explained the sales rep. "In the morning, the key opinion leader would take us into surgery, and he would have three or four patients lined up. We'd watch the doctor show them how to do it; they could scrub in and they could also touch the patient, and things like that. Made them feel comfortable."

Before the sales reps left, they told the physicians that they had to agree to "stack" five patients for surgery. Repetition was the key to success, according to sales reps.

The learning curve for the mesh implants was about three to five cases back-to-back, three as a minimum, J&J sales reps said. If the doctors did only one implant a week, they would "forget" the details. Three back-to-back would help the doctors retain the skill set until they could schedule more mesh implants. Furthermore, it would give the doctors confidence to keep trying. Of course, said the ex–sales rep, women were not to be told that they were only the doctor's third, or second, or even first implant patient.

"They [the doctors] were on their own after that. If they needed us, they would call us," said the sales reps.

But the "low-hanging fruit"—the ob-gyns who lacked hours in surgical training—weren't always able to "stack" patients for operations, and the dearth of experience in such surgery inevitably led to mistakes.

"Look, you have to understand these doctors aren't surgeons to begin with; they're obstetricians, so they're not trained in that space. They didn't do that in residency. And they are doing everything blind, everything by tactile sensation, and by whatever we are telling them," said the ex-rep.

Occasionally, a patient would tell her doctor sometime after the implant that the mesh was poking through her vaginal wall and her partner would complain that it was cutting his penis. "We'd tell the doctor to bring the patient in and trim the mesh off. Send her home with an ice pack" and some estrogen-laced cream to soothe and strengthen the vaginal tissue, said ex-rep.

However, there was one side effect related to the lack of surgical experience that became a problem for many ob-gyns pretty quickly. "The biggest thing was shortening the length of the vagina. That was a big deal," said the ex–sales rep. He was echoed by several doctors who still do, or did, mesh implants—or who make a living trying to repair the damage.

The sales reps said they tried to coax doctors not to go "short," but many ob-gyns didn't push far enough into the vagina to make their incision. They were "scared to go the entire 8 cm length of the vagina." At the apex of the vagina is the recto space. "Ob-gyns were scared to go past the apex, because they didn't want to go into the bladder," said an ex-rep.

The area behind the vaginal wall was traditionally off-limits to ob-gyns. He explained the way the female body below the waist was traditionally parceled out to different doctors. "The bladder belongs to the urologist," he said. And if, during a mid-urethral sling implant, the doctor punctures the urethra, "Well, that belongs to the urologist. They [ob-gyns] can't be messing with it. And the urologist will tell them they shouldn't even have been there to begin with," said the ex-rep.

With that in the background, ob-gyns figured that if they were going to "err, they were going to undercut things, not overcut things." And that's how thousands of women ended up with shortened vaginas—which led to a host of other medical issues including severe pain, infection, worsening incontinence, and painful sex—particularly painful for their husbands.

When companies began selling more complex mesh kits for pelvic organ prolapse, the side effects increased, causing more severe damage. "At that point, doing prolapse, these doctors were repairing the cystocele and rectocele [an operation that lifts and tightens the tissue around the bladder and rectum so these organs no longer push against the vagina], and that was right next to the bladder. And they just don't belong there," said the sales rep.

Many ob-gyn doctors can perform hysterectomies. But that involves the uterus, and the uterus has nothing to do with the urinary tract. "Ob-gyns are not trained in vesicovaginal or rectovaginal space, [i.e.,] what we were trained for," said the ex–sales rep.

"But we convinced them it was a simple procedure and we could walk them through it. They could bill, make money, and start developing to be opinion leaders," said the ex-rep.

"High-volume" doctors would bring in a few more colleagues, who in turn would bring in new recruits. In some respects, it was like Amway and other popular pyramid schemes. "Our job was to convince them how easy it is," said the ex-rep.

There were a number of ways to avoid the poor implant technique, but as former sales reps noted, they all involved proactive moves by companies—some foresight, some funding, and perhaps even slowing down the rush to market while the companies improved the actual implant techniques for the new mesh surgeons.

"Ethicon should have had urologists or pelvic surgeons oversee those first implants the new recruits did on live patients," said former J&J sales reps. "Ethicon could have saved themselves and patients a lot of trouble, a lot of pain, and [the redoing of] surgeries," said the former sales reps.

Lacking enough real proctors, mesh maker sales reps soon found themselves in the role of coach, maybe even colleague. They would help the doctors in the OR, answer their questions about mesh tension, guide the doctor's hand, and show where to place the instrument. And occasionally (more often in private surgery centers than in hospitals), the sales rep's assistance led to the rep touching the patient, the ex-rep acknowledged.

"So the surgeons were placing this mesh in the vesicovaginal and the rectovaginal spaces blindly. They were using tactile sensation, and they were being coached by us."

"We'd say: 'Look, Doctor, what do you feel? I want you to dissect this space using so much of this solution. After you dissect, I want you to go lateral until you feel a certain landmark, keep on going lateral, keep on going laterally until you feel a certain landmark. Now run your hand over this. Do you feel that? Yeah? Okay, let's go ahead and start measuring, and let's start placing the mesh in the vagina.'"

Sometimes the doctors would not dissect properly to get to the right planes; other times they would nick the bladder.

In retrospect, said one of the ex-reps, the program wasn't focused on patients. "We were training ob-gyns because they were the ones referring patients to urologists and urogynecologists—the enemies."

"We thought we could hit the max [recruiting doctors] and hit them all. Low-hanging fruit. Just coach them. It's a simple procedure.

"In doing this, we were harming these women, but we didn't know it at the time," he said.

"I can't believe I got mixed up in this," he ended. "I'm a good guy."

THE SECRET OF NO PLAN B

Behind the scenes, scientists and many in the urogynecologic community had known for years that there were concerns about the most basic part of the implant technique itself, the entry. Going in through the vagina, a non-sterile field, was likely going to affect the mesh implant. Infection was more than a relatively low risk.

Furthermore, the doctors and scientists also knew there were serious questions about the safety and viability of the actual implant material—the mesh. Already, there was data showing the mesh could erode, shrink, or tear after placement inside the patient.

If there was significant "erosion" or, even worse, "migration," it might require surgery to remove or "explant" the mesh implant. And there was nothing in the IFU (instructions for use) leaflet that came with the implant suggesting why or how to remove it. After all, the mesh was supposed to be permanent.

One outside consulting surgeon did attempt to develop an "explant" procedure. But Ethicon didn't want that publicized because it might cause people—doctors or patients—to think some implants might need to be removed.

"I think we should understand more about [the specialist's] technique before encouraging any publication/promotion of his [explant] method," wrote an Ethicon executive on October 3, 2000, to other Ethicon mesh doctors.

She did not like the idea of publicly discussing the "explant." It could feed the competitors' campaigns against TVT. "We must be very careful in avoiding 'over information.'"

She wrote: "Theoretically, I can envision no need for a TVT explant." Then she added, "If we, in any way, publish such information, we start giving the reason to believe that explant of the TVT may be needed in some circumstances."

Finally, she admitted, "Frankly, I do not want to dig my own grave . . . !"

The companies didn't share these issues or these emails with ob-gyns or the public. If doctors asked the sales reps or their "trainers" about potential problems, they got the official companies' talking points:

- Hernia mesh has a terrific track record.
- Vaginal mesh is similar to hernia mesh.
- The implant is safe and has minimal risks.
- It is a much quicker procedure than Burch surgery.
- And, Doctor, it has a hell of a profit margin.

KATRINA'S STORY

Terry doesn't make a habit of chasing doctors or dragging them back to examination rooms. In fact, he'd never done anything like that before that day when he followed a gynecological surgeon at Emory University's prestigious medical school down a hospital hall, and with a nurse, marched the physician back to the exam cubicle where his wife Katrina was starting to sob. "I had to do something. I rushed out and told the nurse, 'Don't let the doctor go. He's got to come back. Now!'"

Katrina was sitting on the exam table, just taking her feet out of the stirrups, wondering why no one except her husband believed her. She couldn't help but wonder that perhaps she really was having a mental breakdown just like her doctors were saying. Terry walked in, almost pulling the doctor along. "I told him, 'You have to examine her again.'" The doctor, who is also a professor at Emory, looked at Terry, then Katrina. He had already spent almost an hour with patient Katrina Spradley.

He'd reviewed about 100 pages of medical records scanning notes from other physicians who'd been treating her the previous five years. The patient claimed to be in constant, almost searing pain. She complained that she felt something inside her. She had frequent urinary and bladder infections that lasted longer and longer. Sometimes she couldn't sit up, couldn't walk. She needed to lose weight, the doctor had told her before he left her room the first time. His orders on the paper given to the nurse said Katrina also should be screened for diabetes and take magnesium tablets to calm her. The doctor could tell she was depressed and upset. Perhaps counseling would help. He couldn't find any mesh protrusion to link to her pain and other symptoms.

"Terry asked the doctor to look inside me again," Katrina says. The doctor, who was "very kind," put on the plastic gloves and said "OK." "Terry stood over the doctor and showed him where to put his hand, how far to go in," Katrina shared in her gentle, soft-spoken way. "The doctor said he still didn't feel anything, and I asked him to go in farther," Terry explains.

And there it was. Poking out of Katrina's vaginal wall, a hardened piece of plastic. The thing that was causing Terry and Katrina so much pain whenever they had relations. Causing Katrina pain every day. The doctor looked up at Terry and Katrina. "It's the mesh," he said, nodding. "Finally!" stated Katrina. "He found it. Was he surprised!" After that moment, a lot happened. The doctor called in other physicians, found the earliest medical records included with Katrina's hysterectomy, and told Katrina he would schedule her for surgery. And, she remarked with a grin on her face, the doctor told her he would never doubt her again.

"It was like the nightmare was finally ending," Katrina exhaled. "It wasn't all in my head."

After so much difficulty getting an accurate diagnosis, let alone treatment, Katrina co-founded a group to help other women in 2018. "Mesh Victims United." Its slogan is simple: "Hope will never be silent." Katrina's story is long and complicated. The short version is that after living with endometriosis for years, Katrina agreed to have a hysterectomy in 2008. She had one child and wasn't planning more. She was 38.

Before her surgery, Katrina mentioned to her doctor that she was starting to have some incontinence when she laughed or sneezed. He said it was a bladder problem that many women experienced after they'd gone through a strenuous childbirth and he could fix it while he was finishing her hysterectomy.

Terry and Katrina had once been high school sweethearts in Georgia. But they'd each married someone else, raised children, and then divorced; now they were back together in Georgia. Katrina had an idea for a new business for the couple, a trucking service. In 2012, they were finishing all the paperwork for the company. Katrina went to truck driving school and finished the requisite lessons. That summer, she had the urine test needed to complete the steps to get her trucker's license. Then she'd gotten the results. There weren't any illicit drugs in her system, but there was blood in her urine. "I'd been having some problems—pain mostly. In my pelvic area, groin, and my vagina," Katrina said. The blood in her urine was a sign that she needed a pelvic exam. But the first physician didn't really find anything. Her symptoms began to worsen. She found herself bouncing from doctor to doctor over the next few years; no one was able to diagnose the cause of her condition.

Finally, around September 2012, Katrina's primary care physician asked if she'd had a mesh implant in her, the stuff that was being used in women to stop them leaking pee. There had been many news reports that year about problems with incontinence and prolapse mesh and several major companies, including Johnson & Johnson, were doing voluntary recalls of some of their popular implant products. Katrina told him she didn't have mesh. "I thought the doctor who did my hysterectomy was tacking up my bladder, with sutures, to stop the incontinence. I didn't realize he was putting in mesh." The primary care physician requested she get her medical records. That very afternoon, the records from the Wisconsin hospital where she had her hysterectomy were faxed to her doctor. And there was the mesh, a transobturator Obtryx made by Boston Scientific.

The primary care doctor quickly referred Katrina to a urology group. The urologists conducted several tests, including scans, and she also had a painful cystoscopy. None of the tests found a source for her pain. In fact, the urologists didn't find the mesh. "I told them I had mesh. They told me it couldn't be 'bad' mesh, because they didn't find it. I told them that Terry had been scratched by it during sex. They said they didn't see mesh."

Terry says, "That so-called scratch takes several days to heal. How did they not find that plastic poking out?" Six months later, Katrina got a referral to a urologist who specialized in pelvic issues at Emory, and that's how she and Terry finally started getting answers.

That doctor at Emory operated several months later and found that the mesh had been disintegrating and locking itself around other organs and nerves. He had to cut what remained of the mesh sling. "I had no bladder control after the sling was removed; I had to wear diapers all the time," says Katrina.

Months later, Katrina and Terry drove to UCLA where Dr. Shlomo Raz, a premier urogynecologist, conducted surgery to remove as much mesh as he could. But, he told her after the procedure, she had a lot of damage that could not be repaired and there was still some mesh in her. Katrina's returned to Dr. Raz for more surgery the next year. "I had rectocele, cystocele—Dr. Raz repaired that—he was terrific—but it was the worst surgery experience."

Because of the damage to the nerves in her leg muscles, Katrina had been getting epidural injections for inflammation and pain in her lower back and hip with local doctors. She limped constantly. Then she had a spinal fluid leak, possibly linked to the pain injections in her spine. A different doctor back in Georgia said he couldn't help her with that pain. "He did not understand what was going on. He wouldn't listen to me. I had all these pelvic problems with the mesh, and from the mesh. The pelvic floor issues were hurting my back, my hips, and these doctors were sending me around to different offices in the same medical building and none of them were talking with each other," Katrina says. Pain and other physical injuries continue to impact Katrina's life. "The damage is done," she says. There may be more medical procedures in the future. The pelvic floor is one of the strongest parts of the body, "but if you start operating on that area it can cause nerve damage and other injuries. I can't push down on my pelvic area for a bowel movement. I have to, but it's hell." "Our lives revolve around the mesh," admits husband Terry. "That's what's so bad. Every day I watch her suffer and deal with it. I go get the buggy for her, take her to the doctor, but I can't take away her pain." Terry's become a dedicated advocate for women hurt by mesh, says Katrina, and he helps with the work she and others are doing through Mesh Victims United to reach other women, give them information, give them a voice—and give them hope. Katrina, who is involved in a suit against the mesh maker, was recently deposed. "The lawyers for the company really pushed me about the group"— why did she found this group? Why is it called Mesh Victims United? What does she intend to do with this group? "I told them it's a non-profit for us women. We've been used to make them money, and tossed aside. We've created a community from what was done to us," Katrina shares.

"I have to accept the fact that I am like this. That makes me a more positive person, so I can help other individuals. I tell the women that they need to be more proactive in their healthcare. It starts there. Ask questions. Demand answers." Katrina's not trucking as much as she was. But she still loves gardening. "I still get out there and crawl on my hands and knees. I don't want to give it up, it's my therapy."

She says, "I wish people understood what it takes to keep me—a person. You know, I'm not even 50 yet."

Katrina's story is one that so many women with vaginal mesh can relate to. It's one of not being told the truth about mesh, not being listened to by doctors who think it's "all in your head", being embarrassed to talk about the difficulties with sex, and feeling guilty for not being able to be the wife, mother, and hard worker that you thought you'd be. It's also one about the struggles of moving on, finding hope, and trying to fix what's broken.

CHAPTER 7

KINGPINS IN THE EXECUTIVE OFFICE

"The people responsible . . . get to walk away with a slap on the wrist. These people are basically very formal drug dealers who are now protected just because they're a corporation. But if you look at someone like El Chapo, what's the major difference? Right? Be like, 'Oh, it's more violent.' Yes, but fundamentally he's a drug dealer. They're all drug dealers. The Feds took his money. Yeah, and he's spending the rest of his life in prison. So, if you think about it, El Chapo really only made one big mistake: he shouldn't have been a drug lord, he should have been the CEO of El Chapo, Inc."

—Trevor Noah

There are three ways to respond if you're a medical device maker and your mesh implant is too complicated for surgeons to implant:

First, you can try to elevate the level of surgeons to whom you sell your device. But focusing on elite doctors would narrow your sales market.

Second, you can radically redesign your mesh device to make it easier to implant without causing additional injuries. But that involves dealing with the FDA, which would inherently result in shutting down the distribution of the product during the FDA intervention. While this makes common sense, the reality is that the medical device manufacturer would be bypassed by competitors in the market for that type of mesh. As a business for profit, this was not an option.

Third, you can advertise your newest mesh product as "easier" to implant, even if surgeons are telling you behind the scenes that it is far too complicated to implant following the directions on its package. You can check back in with doctors later—that's what post-market surveillance is for. This way, you maintain your large market full of less experienced surgeons without losing any revenue. That's basically what Johnson & Johnson did with their extremely lucrative TVT line of incontinence slings.

Johnson & Johnson's Ethicon division and its subsidiary Gynecare had received emails, calls, and reports about unexpected failure rates in mesh surgeries involving the TVT "classic" incontinence sling and its sequel, the TVT-O. The TVT "classic" seemed less prone to serious side effects and failures by the standards of some other slings on the market and in comparison to the TVT-O. Nonetheless, there was a growing number of reports of side effects for incontinence mesh slings, including J&J's.

New mesh doctors had been told that these mesh implants were relatively easy to put in place. In fact, as sales reps and experienced surgeons agreed, the procedure was quite intricate. What *was* easy was the ability to accidentally cause permanent damage to a woman's bladder or urethra, or provoke excessive bleeding. Or all three.

Only skilled surgeons who repeatedly performed vaginal mesh procedures could do the widely promoted "15-minute" drill with the implant and end up with a patient who was "dry" (meaning, stress-induced incontinence was reduced) and not in significant pain two weeks later.

To address those "too complicated" mesh implantations, Ethicon jumped to the forefront of a nascent movement to produce a single-incision sling for incontinence, beating their competitors American Medical Systems and Boston Scientific. In 2006, Ethicon's subsidiary

Gynecare launched a new sling named the TVT-Secur, which became the first of a cadre of industry meshes called "mini-slings."

The TVT-Secur saga became one of the classic "I told you so" moments in this vaginal mesh mania—the problems reported were manifold. (People inside the FDA developed a few pejorative nicknames for different companies' "mini-slings" because of the number of their side effects that just seemed inevitable.)

It generated a dozen or more medical studies over the following decade such as "The Short Life Cycle of a Medical Device."

Similar to the Mentor ObTape fiasco, the TVT-Secur story showed how multinational corporations played with, and relied on, the lack of communication between foreign countries' health agencies and the US Food and Drug Administration. The FDA, which was supposed to protect patients in the prized American sales market, was apparently kept quarantined from negative news from abroad on mesh sling injuries and sales decisions.

BUILT FOR SPEED

There's little question among researchers and many doctors who tried to implant the TVT-Secur that J&J pushed it to market too fast. Johnson & Johnson's marketing chiefs thought the same way as Boston Scientific did in its "Speed to Market Report": You hold on to your market share by promising something new on the horizon, even if your current product is (relatively) good. This will undermine competitors' efforts to cut into your market with "new" and "innovative" products.

Ethicon needed TVT-Secur to recapture its market share and maintain its revenue, so it planned on charging a 15 percent premium (compared to its existing sling products), according to the 2017 medical expert report for lawyers suing J&J. The author, Dr. Ralph Zipper, cited many internal Ethicon documents and emails.

One was written by TVT-Secur's creator, Dan Smith, a biomedical engineer at Ethicon. "Being first to market with a superior less-invasive TVT product and protecting our market share could be priceless," Smith said. It was no surprise that the TVT-Secur launch took priority over clinical trials and data.

But that rush to market worried a number of people inside Ethicon. One was Johnson & Johnson's worldwide group marketing director Harel Gadot. He notified the head of Ethicon's Women's Health & Urology worldwide marketing director of his concerns regarding the plan to skip clinical trials, according to Dr. Zipper's detailed report. "I would strongly recommend to find a way not to cancel completely the proposed RCT (randomized clinical trials)," Gadot wrote. The lack of true clinical data could hurt TVT-Secur's support among Ethicon's key opinion leaders in Europe, such as Professor Carl Nilsson, colleague of the late Ulf Ulmsten.

But the launch was already set.

At times like this, it's important to remind ourselves that a "new and improved" product version is superfluous—New Coke, anyone?

And sometimes it's a fiasco. There was no medical need for a "stiffer" incontinence mesh when Mentor took its ObTape to market. There was only a *marketing* need for Mentor to do something to separate itself from other companies that were already successfully selling thousands of mesh products.

In theory, the concept of the single-incision method seemed perfect. One incision should be simpler to attach through the vagina than earlier sling implants, which required multiple incisions at various locations prior to placement. The novel approach targeted doctors who were less confident and more conservative about taking patients into the operating room.

It was also a good way to recruit ob-gyns who were still referring women with incontinence to urogynecologists. Internal Ethicon documents show that TVT's single-incision method was directly aimed at the non-surgeon doctors the company was recruiting. Sales reps said the single-incision sling instilled "a false sense of security" compared to implanting other slings. But it was really about meeting the procedure quotas among doctors that would get Ethicon the sales numbers they wanted.

TVT-Secur received 510(k) clearance in November 2005, managing to circumvent the FDA's earlier request for one year of clinical data.

Afterward, Ethicon executives sent emails congratulating its team on getting the 510(k) clearance. One praised them for sidestepping "tricky questions raised by the FDA." Another said the fast 510(k) clearance helped Ethicon achieve a "considerable savings of resources, time, and potentially delayed sales."

TVT-Secur went to market in 2006 with the blessing of Wall Street and a handful of sheep and cadaver studies. (In fact, according to Dr. Zipper's 2017 report, Ethicon tested TVT-Secur's mesh fixation implement using TVTx—a product similar to TVT-Secur, but without the same fixation barb—in its live sheep lab. The actual TVT-Secur fixation was tested in sheep cadavers.)

Gynecare quickly began receiving reports about complications from, among other countries, Germany and Australia. The surgical instructions were poorly defined, many doctors said.

In addition, there was a longer-than-anticipated learning curve; the company had projected five cases to bring a doctor up to the skills needed for implant. It actually needed at least 15 to 20 cases, according to one of Ethicon's top consultants, Dr. Menahem Neuman.

Sales of TVT-Secur did not hit their target of $25.5 million the first year, but they did reach $21.47 million. At the time of TVT-Secur's official launch in 2006, its main rivals were the AMS MiniArc and the Boston Scientific Prefyx.

Despite the pile of reports that surgery for TVT-Secur was a difficult procedure well beyond many doctors' skill levels, Ethicon kept marketing the mesh to doctors and patients as simple and less invasive.

THE FLYING SURGEONS

When Ethicon mobilized for battle with its competitors, it did not skimp on resources. Its shipment of high-volume urogynecologists to Sweden to learn mesh implants from the master, Ulf Ulmsten, was only the first of its global flight program.

As its TVT line piled up revenue in the US, the company mobilized a number of private surgeons and sent them to Europe and elsewhere to start teaching implants of their single-incision, polypropylene TVT-Secur.

The teams had acquired a nickname from sales reps and some of the doctors: the Flying Surgeons. Their role, in addition to conducting training sessions abroad, was to report back on TVT-Secur's acceptance level by doctors in other countries and to voice any problems they encountered.

That's what Dr. Menahem Neuman did in 2007 in a memorable PowerPoint for Ethicon on "The European Flying Surgeon" adventure with TVT-Secur. Dr. Neuman, who is based in Israel, ticked off appallingly high failure rates for TVT surgery. He cited the lack of appropriate training among doctors trying out the implant. The TVT-Secur program needed more expert key opinion leaders to participate in training programs.

Neuman's slides warned the learning curve was not three to four procedures, but really "25–30 operations before a 'surgeon's maturity.'" That number was not going to be met by Johnson & Johnson's weekend trainees.

In an interview for this book, Dr. Neuman said the various mini-slings were problematic because of their design. "Too complex for any but skilled surgeons to implant," he said. "I did 1,004 TVT-Secur procedures, 7,000 TVT procedures in all. The success rate of the mini-slings—all the companies'—was not that high," he said.

The first problem was the lack of skill among the doctors recruited by companies to implant the mini-slings and the poorly drafted instructions for use, he said. The second was the mesh—there was too much of it, and it was too wide.

That problem was soon exacerbated with the arrival of prolapse kits. "It's like American cars—you want the largest," he commented. "I was persuaded at the time that these newer implants would work, but we didn't really know. There were no clinical trials."

He added, "That was a big mistake; the company was very arrogant."

Dr. Neuman said, "We should treat implants like medications—the smaller the dose, the fewer side effects. And you must have proper clinical trials before you dare to include implants into your practice."

Neuman's "Flying Surgeon" PowerPoint ended with a picture of a little boy and his dog at bedtime. The little boy was kneeling, his eyes tightly closed as he was praying. The slide said "TVT-Secur—The First 265 Operations." Asked what that meant, Dr. Neuman said that people were praying TVT-Secur would work.

SHOW ME THE MONEY!

In August 2007, Ethicon/Gynecare's WW (Worldwide) Marketing Team for Women's Health & Urology unveiled a plan for world domination of the female incontinence mesh market.

They had created a slideshow for people on Ethicon's Incontinence Platform. It began with a photo from the movie *Jerry Maguire.* Actor Tom Cruise was standing with Cuba Gooding Jr. during the moment in the movie when the NFL player portrayed by Gooding demands that his agent, played by Cruise, deliver the lucrative contract he was promised. Gooding's immortal line is "SHOW ME THE MONEY!" The slide put it up all in capitals.

The show quickly got into the "Total TVT Family" in sales globally. TVT was in Canada, Europe, the Middle East, Asia Pacific, and Latin America. The US had the largest market. The slides shouted: "WE STRENGTHEN OUR POSITION AS THE MARKET LEADER IN 2007. We are gaining back market share. We are growing the category."

Then came a litany of issues surrounding TVT-Secur. Apparently, TVT-O—the Obturator—was the "preferable approach," not the newer Secur sling.

There was a "big deviation in satisfaction" among current users regarding TVT-Secur.

The slideshowed a list of the "main difficulties/complications" including:

1. Insertion difficulties
2. Releasing difficulties
3. Fixation tips not staying in place
4. Bladder perforation

5. Excessive bleeding
6. **FAILURES—Tensioning**

"Not-well-defined 'cookbook' instructions procedure leads to differences in the technique between surgeons," said the next slide. The learning curve took "much longer" than originally anticipated, and doctors likely needed to do 15–20 cases instead of five to become very comfortable with TVT-Secur.

And some "customers" (doctors) refused to do training sessions on TVT-Secur. They were "know-all surgeons," chided the slide. According to the PowerPoint, two surgeons who had been among the first in Europe to try TVT-Secur were "not supporting" the product.

Finally, there was a lack of real testing. "Other leading KOLs insist on clinical data first," read the slide. That must have been a disappointment.

To address this list of issues, Ethicon/Gynecare was going to see that the procedural "cookbook" was standardized, with emphasis on "hands-on training." They would establish clinical data, obtain new KOLs to advocate for TVT-Secur, set up a cadaver lab, and send top Ethicon medical experts to personally visit some European sites "to assist in overcoming difficulties" in Germany and France. And for this campaign to save TVT-Secur, they would turn to their five "experienced flying surgeons."

The slideshow moved on to "Meet the Flintstones." On one side was a photo of a sling going into a vagina. On the other was a cartoon of Fred Flintstone in a prehistoric operating cave, holding a car wrench, presumably doing a Burch procedure. This point was "sling surgery versus traditional surgery" for incontinence. "Project Flintstone" would drag cave dwellers into the modern world, where SUI surgery took only as long as the drive-thru line at Dairy Queen.

The goal was to convert traditionalists to mesh. The company would enroll would-be implanters in six areas—Italy, the Middle East, Egypt, Germany, Greece, and Russia. These places accounted for 72 percent of all traditional procedures across the European–North African area. A "lack of education" was cited as the reason for so many doctors still doing SUI the old-fashioned way. Ethicon would offer training in implants—an anatomy course, a cadaver lab, and live "hands-on" surgery. The kickoff for the TVT campaign would be October 10, to "capitalize on the 10-year mark since the launch of classic TVT."

As early as October 2007, internal Ethicon emails shared that one doctor reported having "a 30% failure rate up to and including his first 77 patients and a 40% failure rate in his first 25." In November 2007, the reported numbers were even worse in Australia as cited between Dr. Aran Maree to Catherine V. Beath, the VP of quality assurance.

"Our initial inquiries indicate that the following are roughly the 6-week success rates for these surgeons:

Prof Malcolm Frazer Performed: ~20 cases, Failure: ~13 cases (he has performed about 700 TVT cases over the years)

Dr. Bruce Farnsworth Performed: ~ 20 + cases, Failure: ~6 cases

Prof Marcus Carey Performed: ~ 20 cases, Failure: "lots of early failures" (8 at least and still counting), awaiting a final number from this surgeon

All of these surgeons have indicated that their success rate with TVT-Secur is substantially below their success rates with TVT-O . . . In short, some of our customers are indicating their concern and a loss of confidence in this product."

And the numbers weren't good in 2008, just one year later. Many doctors were complaining about trying to determine the right tension of the sling with prior models, which made this new version appealing. However, internal emails between Harel Gadot to Price St. Hilaire, two of Ethicon's marketing managers, stated, "It took us a few months to clear the right placement of the mesh with all of our customers, but many of them feel uncomfortable with the final placement due to the problems with releasing the device . . . What (and why) is the right tension. We did cover this in the new Prof. Ed. CD, but I believe we need to take it a step further."

CHAPTER 8

DOWN UNDER . . . THE SILENT RECALL

"There were clearly problems with TVT-Secur from the beginning. We planned for 50 patients, and we closed the trial at 28 because of all the problems we already saw."

—Dr. Malcolm Frazer

There was Ethicon, prepping for a big anniversary celebration, an occasion to propel their mesh sales and salvage the reputation of TVT-Secur.

But down under in Australia, doctors weren't in the mood to light candles on a cake. They wanted to start a bonfire, built of TVT-Secur kits. And one of the people holding a torch worked for the company.

Ex–Ethicon sales reps talk about what happened as though it were a legendary battle in *Game of Thrones.*

"There was this guy, his name was Maree," said one former rep. "I don't know if this is one of the most honest guys in the health-care industry, or if he'd just had such a backlash that he had to do something about it, but he started blowing the whistle on TVT-Secur, and getting real hot with Ethicon over the failure rate there—it was maybe 30 percent.

"That is why Australia did what we call the silent recall. Doctors here didn't know anything about it," said the ex-rep. "But a lot of people at Ethicon were copied on his emails."

Aran Maree. A graduate of the Royal College of Surgeons in Dublin, Maree joined Johnson & Johnson in Sydney in 2006. He was the head of Medical Devices for ANZ (Australia and New Zealand) and head of Strategic Medical Affairs for that territory. And he's been a volunteer for the North Bondi Beach SLSC—Surf Life Saving Club—since 1998.

> "I want to just reiterate my concerns regarding the high 'failure' rates across multiple centres that we are seeing with TVT-Secur when compared to its predecessor TVT-O. I feel that you should be aware of our issues with TVT-Secur for your surveillance in other AP countries and in case there are aspects on which you may have any further advice for me."

On October 24, 2007, the head of medical affairs in Women's Health at Ethicon, Price St. Hilaire, sent messages to Ethicon executives in other countries about a review of TVT-Secur issues completed by the US "team" with 25 preceptors, the consulting doctors who had been training and overseeing Ethicon mesh implants in America.

St. Hilaire said 100 percent of the preceptors wanted an "improved release mechanism" for the TVT-Secur and a "reduced inserter profile." In other words, the release on the TVT-Secur that should allow the mesh to set into place did not function easily at times and the "inserter" tool was too large. St. Hilaire wanted to know if Ethicon preceptors or executives saw any similar problems identified in the US.

Indeed they did. Dr. Maree was already reading about "complaints" from surgeons comparing the TVT-Secur unfavorably with Ethicon's TVT-O (and the TVT-O was not problem-free itself).

On October 25, Maree sent a couple "HIGHLY CONFIDENTIAL" emails to other Asia-Pacific-based Ethicon doctors and then to others up the chain. He was blunt: "I want to just reiterate my concerns regarding the high 'failure' rates across multiple centres that we are seeing with TVT-Secur when compared to its predecessor TVT-O. I feel that you should be aware of our issues with TVT-Secur for your surveillance in other AP countries and in case there are aspects on which you may have any further advice for me."

Maree said, "While we launched in Australia just under 12 months ago, we have not yet launched this product in New Zealand," making it clear that he didn't want to move too fast with TVT-Secur.

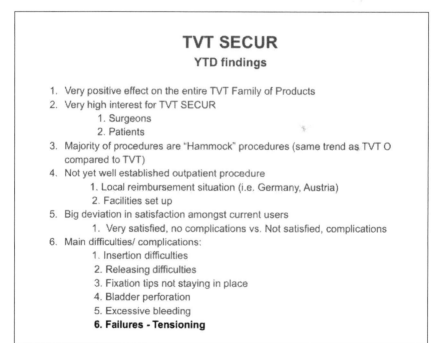

TVT SECUR
YTD findings

1. Very positive effect on the entire TVT Family of Products
2. Very high interest for TVT SECUR
   1. Surgeons
   2. Patients
3. Majority of procedures are "Hammock" procedures (same trend as TVT O compared to TVT)
4. Not yet well established outpatient procedure
   1. Local reimbursement situation (i.e. Germany, Austria)
   2. Facilities set up
5. Big deviation in satisfaction amongst current users
   1. Very satisfied, no complications vs. Not satisfied, complications
6. Main difficulties/ complications:
   1. Insertion difficulties
   2. Releasing difficulties
   3. Fixation tips not staying in place
   4. Bladder perforation
   5. Excessive bleeding
   6. **Failures - Tensioning**

Maree cited numbers involving three TVT-experienced doctors in Australia who were seeing "failure" rates of 25–50 percent. They were having issues with the instructions for implant.

The IFU had been reviewed by one of Ethicon's top preceptors and consultants, Dr. Vincent Lucente. He was a leading urogynecologist and skilled surgeon in Pennsylvania and among the "high-volume" mesh implant specialists. Lucente reported a high success rate with TVT-Secur using the instructions. But many other doctors had not.

"I have had uncorroborated verbal feedback only to the effect that Dr. Lucente has subsequently had to modify his technique from the original training to improve his results somewhat, but that his 'failure rate' may still be higher than with TVT-O," wrote Maree. He noted that the Australian doctor Malcolm Frazer, whom he knew, had adopted Lucente's "modified technique." But Frazer "is not experiencing a substantial improvement in success rates."

Maree said, "My concerns are the following: this product may have been launched as a substitute for TVT-O without enough clinical data to justify such a rollout.

"The original (and current?) training program may not result in competency in device insertion or result in clinical efficacy," he continued. "There appear to be 'tricks' to insertion of the product and removal of the inserters which prevent dislodging the device in the process, etc.

"As a company, we need to ensure that we protect the good name of J&J's reputation and avoid such issues going forward elsewhere with this product and with other products." Maree said that his team was reporting the complaints "through correct channels" to Gynecare. They would also have to make a report to Australian regulators, "since 3 patients (so far) have required re-operation at this stage."

Then he invoked the company's ethics pledge, its "credo," which signaled how worried he was. Maree said that with the credo as guidance, Johnson & Johnson had the "responsibility to ensure that we are diligent as a company in performing an adequate pre-market assessment on multiple dimensions before launching a new product."

He wrote, "We will also need to check that new products, when either significantly modified from predecessors or which bring with them a substantially new technique, have adequate pre-market safety and efficacy clinical data to justify their launch."

Maree alluded to another important point: The threat of more demands from various government health authorities for testing if

Ethicon didn't find the cause of the TVT-Secur problem and show they were fixing it. "Otherwise, we will merely force [regulators] to require a higher level of clinical evidence for every new product, even where arguably not justified."

In one exchange, Maree said, "While I do not want to appear unnecessarily negative about what I am sure is a well-designed and innovative product, I know that (others in Australia) with whom I regularly discuss our adverse events, may well suggest that this device may be more successful on the drawing board than in reality, because the average practitioner finds it too complicated to insert correctly or cannot master the process."

From: HARKNESS, Darryl [MEDAU]

Sent: Tue, 30 Oct 2007 00:55:15 GMT

To: MAREE, Aran [MEDAU] <amaree@MEDAU.jnj.com>

Subject: Re: SEDCUR Update presented in at WW Mktg Meeting

Hi, Aran, can you please advise the timing for this phone link as I would like to join. Thanks Darryl

---

Sent using BlackBerry

---------Original Message---------
From: MAREE, Aran [MEDAU]
To: GRIEBEL, Paul [MEDAU] : LAW, Jan [MEDAU]
CC: BUDDEN, Laurie [MEDAU] : CAPPLIS, Anne [MEDAU]: FORAGE, Jenny [MEDAU]:
HARKNESS, Darryl [MEDAU]: Kboo, Teng Chaan Dr. [MEDAP]
Sent: Tue Oct 30 10:14:33 2007
Subject: FW: SECUR Update presented in at WW Mktg Meeting

Dear Paul and Jan,

Thanks for sending this through. The slide deck below had not been sent to me yet and it is quite illuminating. I have cut and pasted the table of Dr. - 6 week outcomes from the slide deck as it is quite striking. In essence he has had a 30% failure rate up to and including his first 77 patients and a 40%failure rate in his first 25. In this light, and given that he was involved in training Dr. Australia, it is not at all surprising that we may have similar, or higher, failure rates here. This is very different to the QA database numbers sent through from the 'reported' complaint rates divided by the USA sales earlier on.

The deck alludes to a 'trick' of Dr. which he is using to improve outcomes and also to 'retraining' or 'expert training' in the use of the device. It also notes that some key KOLs, involved in the first European studies, are refusing to use this device until there is more clinical data.

<<ole0.bemp>>

We need to discuss this deck in detail with David and Joe at our telecon tomorrow night, but as a team, we also need to make some important decisions in the near future regarding the use of this product in Australia.

(i) Who is responsible for monitoring the impact of this product and its success or failure on Australia patients (who were previously well served by TVT O)
(ii) Are we confident that 'retraining' is useful and will truly improve outcomes with TVT Secur? Does retraining work? Are there truly any good datasets there which give us confidence that we can get an acceptable level of No SUI? Is it truly possible to get to the 92% success rate now (apparently) seen by Dr.
(iii) Who with and when will we go ahead with retraining if this is our decision?
(iv) Do we stop further roll-out of this product until our three high volume initial users reach an acceptable level of success? What is this level?
(v) Should we cease to market this product in Australia until we have objective evidence which gives us

"In this case, if some surgeons cannot achieve competency early on, we should restrict access to those who can."

Such a suggestion might rule out recruiting ob-gyns to part-time pelvic surgery. But it was far too late to stop that, at least in the US.

MENTOR REDUX

That email triggered responses across the Australia–New Zealand territory and beyond, quickly bouncing up the chain. Within a couple of days there were about a dozen people on different message lines from Down Under to New Jersey.

Some Ethicon execs seemed to feel that Maree was overreacting; they also wanted to ensure that the mesh itself was not identified as the problem, only the doctors putting it in. Perhaps revising training of the surgeons would work.

> "In this case, if some surgeons cannot achieve competency early on, we should restrict access to those who can."

Formally changing the wording for the instructions for use might mean that the US FDA would have to be notified. This would lead to the agency having to approve changes to those instructions and then someone would have to explain to the FDA what had gone amiss that had led to revisions in the directions for putting in the sling.

Meanwhile, Dr. Lucente had developed some "tricks" while doing the surgical procedure that might ameliorate problems with the stubborn placement mechanism or that might regulate the tension of the tension-free TVT-Secur sling implant.

Perhaps just letting surgeons know about Dr. Lucente's "tricks" and other variations, and informally telling surgeons that some doctors like Lucente were achieving a good "success" rate—and "retraining" some of them—might suffice.

On November 2, 2007, Dr. Maree dropped a bomb on Ethicon's worldwide VP for risk and quality assessment. In a lengthy email to Catherine Beath, Maree said the situation with TVT-Secur was so uncertain that he had made an appointment for November 9 to talk with the Australian regulatory authority for medical devices about reports on "patient adverse events."

In fact, he noted, there had already been a meeting in Paris in May about "issues" experienced by surgeons with TVT-Secur.

Then Maree proposed the "most appropriate customer-focused and credo-aligned position" to take with TVT-Secur in the Australian market: "We feel that withdrawing the product from the market here is currently the most appropriate action for Australia."

The rapid response from the US suggested there was no need to act prematurely.

Ethicon was apparently concerned that if Australia's Ethicon offices pulled TVT-Secur, it could trigger other actions and reactions globally. For instance, could a "safety alert" announced in Australia have ramifications in other parts of the world? Perhaps in the US?

Company chiefs in New Jersey told Maree they would begin a thorough quality investigation, but it could take time.

It's uncertain what exactly Ethicon US expected Maree to do.

But around the beginning of November, Aran Maree imposed a "quality hold" on TVT-Secur. That much is known, because in 2013 Maree was deposed in the 100,000-claim federal tort case against Johnson & Johnson and asked what he did and why.

"If a quality block is put on, no warehouse employee can release a product," Maree explained in his deposition. The company's IT system would prevent any further sales. That of course stalled any future release of TVT-Secur in New Zealand as well.

Prodded a little by the plantiffs' attorney, Maree confirmed in his testimony that he imposed the quality block because of "efficacy and safety" concerns.

J&J's own director of safety for medical devices in Australia and New Zealand had effectively produced a "silent recall."

There were no national news releases Down Under or warnings from the corporation to the public in that immediate time frame of November–December 2007. TVT-Secur just was not available there.

Were US FDA officials told about Australia's silent recall—the "quality block"? Maree said he didn't notify them and that he was "not sure" if the company had known.

Let's pause here for a moment. Ethicon US clearly knew about this recall in Australia. Furthermore, the product wasn't discontinued from the US market—yes, discontinued, not recalled—until March 2013. During its time on the market, 1,647 adverse events were reported and many more went unreported. Ethicon, doctors, and the FDA clearly knew that this product was injuring thousands of American women, but it was not recalled. How is it that Australian women were protected, but not those in the US? Americans pride ourselves on freedom, equality, and innovation, and yet concerning mesh, Australia has been on the cutting edge in many ways. We can only imagine how many women could have been spared the nightmare of mesh if Ethicon had made this an international recall or if the American officials and medical agencies had taken action years sooner.

362
Ross S1, Ducey A2, Robert M2
1.University of Alberta, **2**. University of Calgary

ASSOCIATION OF ADVERSE EVENT REPORTING WITH DISCONTINUATION OF A SURGICAL DEVICE: THE CASE OF TVT SECUR VERSUS TVT-O FOR TREATMENT OF STRESS URINARY INCONTINENCE IN WOMEN

Hypothesis / aims of study

Gynecare TVT Secur ™ (Gynecare, Ethicon Inc., Somerville, MA, USA) was the first commercial single-incision mini-sling device available in Europe and North America for the surgical treatment of stress urinary incontinence. The device was first marketed in 2006 and discontinued for commercial reasons in March 2013. We undertook a comprehensive review of the published literature on TVT Secur [1] to explore the events leading to the withdrawal of TVT Secur. At the same time, we became aware that adverse events were being reported on the MAUDE database. The MAUDE system in the USA includes reports of medical device adverse events that are submitted by the FDA by mandatory reporters (manufacturers, importers and device user facilities) and voluntary reporters such as healthcare professionals, patients and consumers in the USA. The database includes details of individual adverse events and can be searched by brand name. Similar reporting schemes are available in other countries such as Canada, Australia and European countries, but are not as easy to search.

The aims of ur current study were to review the MAUDE database to explore the year and type for TVT Secur compared to TVT-O ™ (Gynecare, Ethicon Inc., Somerville, MA. USA), with particular interest in the date of withdrawal of TVT Secur.

Study design, materials and methods

A retrospective review was undertaken of the adverse events appearing in the MAUDE database from 2007 (shortly after the introduction of TVT Secur) to the end of 2014(21 months after the withdrawal of TVT Secur). Data were collected for each adverse event report for TVT Secur (the device of interest). Data were also collected for TVT-O as a comparison device produced by the same manufacturer during the same time interval. For each device was collated by year.

Results

Over the period of interest, there were 1647 adverse event reports for TVT Secur, versus 18 for TVT-O. Only 3 of these reports were for malfunctions (2 for TVT Secur and 1 for TVT-O). In the period before the withdrawal of TVT Secur (pre 2013), there were 18 adverse events reported for TVT Secur, and 14 for TVT-O. The majority (1530/1647, 91%) of the TVT Secur reports appeared in 2013, the year of the device's withdrawal, peaking at 369 reports in August 2013. In the second half of 2014, the rate of adverse event reports for TVT Secur dropped to 3/month.

Interpretation of results

Our study explored adverse events reported for TVT Secur versus TVT-O over the period including the discontinuation of TVT Secur for commercial reasons. Taking into consideration the probable lower volume of TVT Secur devices implanted over the period before 2013 compared to those reported for TVT-O devices. It seems that the actual number of adverse events likely represents a higher incidence rate of adverse events associated with TVT Secur. The Huge spike in the number of adverse event reports in the noths immediately after TVT Secur was disconnected seems to be associated with reports by attorneys, or instigated by attorneys but reported by others. Our research is seeking further details about the types of individuals reporting adverse events, and about the types of adverse events are reported.
The main advantage of the MAUDE database is that it can be searched by product name, so it was easy to identify the relevant adverse event reports. However, our study also highlights some of the challenges associated with using the MAUDE database for research. A particular problem is the lack of a denominator. We are unable to access the total number of devices either sold for research. A particular problem is lack of denominator. We are unable to access the total number of devices either sold or implanted Data are unlikely ever to be made available, even to the company (in this case Gynecare). We cannot therefore report the risk of adverse events associated with each device. As well, adverse events are often reported years after women have their index surgery, because the event may occur long after the surgery, or else because an adverse event may not be recognized by women as a problem that could be associated with their surgery. In addition, the reports may be duplicated if reported on different dates from different sources.

While Ethicon people were discussing what would happen in the event of an actual "safety alert," which would "require FDA notification as well," tens of thousands of American women were thrown into the battleground of integrity versus profitability.

If you're having déjà vu, you are not alone. Yes, these actions by Ethicon's corporate leadership in the US almost mimic Mentor's move to keep a lid on the serious problems in France about its ObTape and the pressure from the government there.

In fact, it's somewhat similar to the situation with the diet-drug duo fen-phen after phentermine and Redux were voluntarily withdrawn. Internal company documents slowly surfaced showing that Wyeth's marketing division had been driving the decision-making about their diet drugs' safety issues—how to fix them, and how much to let America's doctors, medical associations, and the FDA know about the extent of the problems. Knowledge isn't just power; it's also *money.*

PICKING UP THE PIECES

Ethicon scrambled to control the TVT-Secur situation in Australia. Maree met with government regulators. He sidestepped Ethicon suggestions that "re-training" doctors might mean TVT-Secur could return to Australia's market, citing regulators' concerns.

Ethicon sent TVT-Secur's inventor, engineer Dan Smith, to Australia to talk with some of the surgeons who had expressed the most concern about TVT-Secur. Smith was going to review implantation techniques and issues about the IFU on where the implant was placed. Perhaps Ethicon US still hoped to get TVT-Secur out of the warehouses and back on the market in Sydney.

But in a lengthy email on November 12, Maree wrote about the backlash from Dr. Frazer in the wake of Dan Smith's visit. "Regarding re-training on key points, Prof Frazer said that he disagreed with the company calling it re-training," Maree's message read.

"This isn't re-training," he quoted Frazer saying. Frazer had told Maree, "This is how things always should have been done and how we always should have been trained."

Also, Frazer said, "The nuances I have been learning in the last two weeks were never what I was taught in the beginning" about TVT-Secur.

And the "re-training" plan might not work anyway. "Prof Frazer is not yet convinced that even with these changes the device is going to be as successful as TVT-O and TVT-Retropubic (classic)," wrote Maree.

Professor Frazer told Maree, "I haven't yet seen enough evidence. Even Vince Lucente's data isn't yet convincing to me."

In an interview for this book, Dr. Malcolm Frazer says he has no problem recalling the TVT-Secur controversy. "It was rushed to market" without testing in humans, among other issues, he said. "They shouldn't even have called the Secur a TVT—it wasn't like their other TVT meshes."

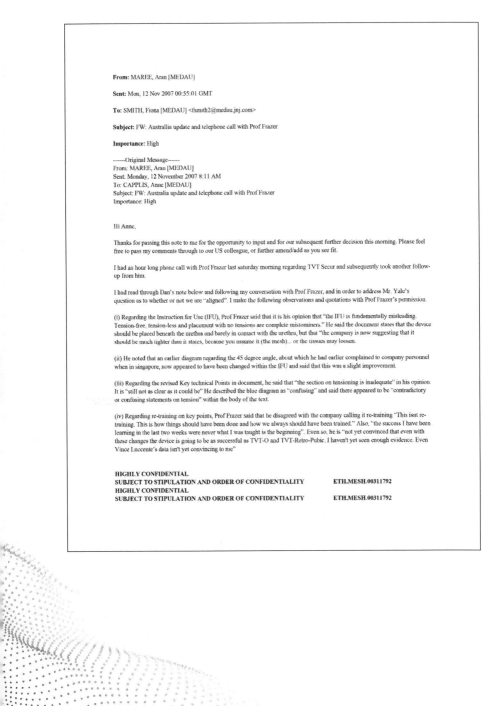

From: MAREE, Aran [MEDAU]

Sent: Mon, 12 Nov 2007 00:55:01 GMT

To: SMITH, Fiona [MEDAU] <fsmith2@medau.jnj.com>

Subject: FW: Australlia update and telephone call with Prof Frazer

Importance: High

------Original Message------
From: MAREE, Aran [MEDAU]
Sent: Monday, 12 November 2007 8:11 AM
To: CAPPLIS, Anne [MEDAU]
Subject: FW: Australia update and telephone call with Prof Frazer
Importance: High

Hi Anne,

Thanks for passing this note to me for the opportunity to input and for our subsequent further decision this morning. Please feel free to pass my comments through to our US colleague, or further amend/add as you see fit.

I had an hour long phone call with Prof Frazer last saturday morning regarding TVT Secur and subsequently took another follow-up from him.

I had read through Dan's note below and following my conversation with Prof Frazer, and in order to address Mr. Yale's question as to whether or not we are "aligned". I make the following observations and quotations with Prof Frazer's permission.

(i) Regarding the Instruction for Use (IFU), Prof Frazer said that it is his opinion that "the IFU is fundamentally misleading. Tension-free, tension-less and placement with no tensions are complete mistommers." He said the document states that the device should be placed beneath the urethra and barely in contact with the urethra, but that "the company is now suggesting that it should be much tighter than it states, because you assume it (the mesh)... or the tissues may loosen."

(ii) He noted that an earlier diagram regarding the 45 degree angle, about which he had earlier complained to company personnel when in singapore, now appeared to have been changed within the IFU and said that this was a slight improvement.

(iii) Regarding the revised Key technical Points in document, he said that "the section on tensioning is inadequate" in his opinion. It is "still not as clear as it could be" He described the blue diagram as "confusing" and said there appeared to be "contradictory or confusing statements on tension" within the body of the text.

(iv) Regarding re-training on key points, Prof Frazer said that he disagreed with the company calling it re-training "This isnt re-training. This is how things should have been done and how we always should have been trained." Also, "the success I have been learning in the last two weeks were never what I was taught is the beginning". Even so, he is "not yet convinced that even with these changes the device is going to be as successful as TVT-O and TVT-Retro-Pubic. I haven't yet seen enough evidence. Even Vince Luccente's data isn't yet convincing to me"

HIGHLY CONFIDENTIAL
SUBJECT TO STIPULATION AND ORDER OF CONFIDENTIALITY   ETH.MESH.00311792
HIGHLY CONFIDENTIAL
SUBJECT TO STIPULATION AND ORDER OF CONFIDENTIALITY   ETH.MESH.00311792

(v) Dan's note that Prf Frazer's initial placement was "in the wrong tissue plain, additionally it was most likely located in the pelvic floor not against the pubic bone and tape tension that was too loose. He performed two Secur "U" and afterwards we spoke and both patients were dry after surgery. He wished to wait 6+ weeks to assess their condition before making any further comments. No "H" was done only "U", does seem to concur with what Prof Frazer indicated to me were the learning he took away from his meeting with dan. However, he has now indicated that his one of the two patients he performed with Dan as part of the training session is currently in urinary retention and is self-catheterising. We will need to report this through the QA database.

(vi) Prof Frazer indicated that before Dan's training visit last week he had been trained on this device by Dr Carey. He mentioned that Dr. Carey and he are sharing initial data on their results and that Dr. Carey has "emailed me indicating a similarly low 55% initial success rate." I am therefore not quite sure what to make of Dan's comment below whichh seems to imply that Dr. Carey only suspended the procedures when he learned of Prof Frazer's poor results.

(vii) I did call Dan to personally discuss any relevant information he may have gleaned from Dr. Carey after speaking to him about his time with Prof Frazer, but when I reached him he was with the Carey family and it would have been inappropriate to have the discussion. I take it from the note below that he hopes to spend time with Dr. Carey in theatre later this week. Please ensure, Anne, that any comments sent back to the USA direct by Dan and which may be permanit under our local regulatory system are fed back to you.

(viii) Prof Frazer also noted that he was now concerned that as he was involved in training of this product in Taiwan, there might be and issue there also which needed to be addressed through the correct channels. Please feed this back to WW Risk Management for their consideration.

Prof Frazer said that he still thinks Ethicon "docs uro-gyne better than other companies" but that TVT Secur is so "utterly different to the other TVT's that it probably shouldn't be called a TVT and the speed of market and breadth of the launch did not take this into account, thus requirering all this subsequent follow-up activity Prof Frazer said he would be delighted to take a call from the company if anyone wished to discuss this with him further and that he will await our response to this matter with interest.

Kind Regards,

Aran

------Original Message------
From: CAPPLIS, Anne [MEDAU]
Sent: Friday, 9 November 2007 10:08 PM
To: MAREE, Aran [MEDAU]
Subject: FW: Australia update

FYI

"I and several colleagues really had the impression that Johnson & Johnson wanted to go head-to-head with American Medical Systems, because AMS was taking part of their market share. They moved too quickly," he said.

"There were clearly problems with TVT-Secur from the beginning," Dr. Frazer added. He and other surgeons had organized a two-hospital prospective trial. "We planned for 50 patients, and we closed the trial at 28 because of all the problems we already saw."

Ethicon might have avoided many of these problems—saving patients pain, permanent injuries to organs or nerves, and money—if it had conducted a clinical trial in live women before it sold the implant.

In October 2007, the company assessed the "lessons learned" from the TVT-Secur experience, according to a review of Ethicon documents by lawyers for plaintiffs. Among those lessons cited were "consider

"There were clearly problems with TVT-Secur from the beginning," Dr. Frazer added. He and other surgeons had organized a two-hospital prospective trial. "We planned for 50 patients, and we closed the trial at 28 because of all the problems we already saw."

not carrying out a first human trial and launching the product at the same time (the learnings from a first human trial should be gathered, digested, and the device/training adjusted accordingly before launch)."

As with the earlier reference to Mentor's actions in France, that may also seem similar to the reader. Remember the post-ProteGen pledge at Boston Scientific? Something about "Do clinical trials in women before you sell the mesh."

It had happened again. And the mesh saga had several more years to go.

CHAPTER 9

BEST HIGH IN TOWN

"I am currently involved in getting a patient to the OR
who had an anterior and posterior Prolift implanted
by another physician. She will likely lose any coital
function as her vaginal length is now 3 cm, and there
is mesh extruding literally everywhere. Also there is
a large stone in the bladder from a bladder perforation with the anterior arm . . . This patient will have a
permanently destroyed vagina, and I am only hoping to get her out of this without more morbidity."

—Email about Prolift to Ethicon from a physician, February 2009

"You can implant the mesh in the time it takes
to order a Domino's pizza" went the sales reps'
script, boasting that this surgery could be performed in 30 minutes or less. "You can do
three or four of these implants in a morning
and still be on the golf course by noon."

—Former Johnson & Johnson sales representative

The year 2007 was a very busy time for Johnson & Johnson's Women's
Health division. They were fending off complaints from Australian,
European, and US doctors who weren't happy with TVT-Secur, while

simultaneously planning global domination of the female incontinence market through the TVT vaginal mesh slings that had prompted those complaints.

It was also the year that the FDA found out that J&J had been selling a new mesh implant for women's pelvises without first clearing it with the agency. Ethicon began marketing its first prolapse or POP kit, called Prolift, in 2005, under the FDA's nose. The FDA generally heard of this when it learned that Ethicon was trying to get fast-track clearance for its planned Prolift + M implant to treat prolapse.

> It's difficult to understand how the nation's medical product safety regulators were not aware that one of the largest companies they oversaw, Johnson & Johnson, was selling a vaginal mesh kit without it going through the usual FDA approval process.

The positive angle here is that unlike many other companies' mesh, Prolift did not cite the infamous ProteGen as its predicate device. Instead, as a predicate, the company cited its own device, Prolift. That set off—according to a former agency official—a surprised reaction within the FDA as device center employees asked what a Prolift was.

The details available to the public of this somewhat-embarrassing event are sketchy at best. The FDA doctor who led the agency section on ob-gyn medical devices, Dr. Colin Pollard, did not respond to repeated requests for comment for this book.

It's difficult to understand how the nation's medical product safety regulators were not aware that one of the largest companies they oversaw, Johnson & Johnson, was selling a vaginal mesh kit without it going through the usual FDA approval process. National vaginal mesh sales across the industry were increasing rapidly, and the agency was certainly aware that mesh products were highly profitable, hyped by Wall Street, and being updated almost constantly for FDA review.

By FDA standards, the agency reacted strongly to the discovery of Prolift on the market. There were phone calls, emails, conversations, and angry letters. The company continued selling Prolift.

Company documents show that J&J/Ethicon had initially intended to formally apply to the FDA for "clearance" using the 510(k) fast-track approval process. But American Medical Systems had beaten J&J to market with its Apogee and Perigee POP kits, winning FDA clearance in 2004. Therefore, J&J/Ethicon was in a panic and rushing to start selling their own version to compete. If they moved quickly enough, maybe they could at least beat Boston Scientific.

Johnson & Johnson defended its sales of Prolift without previous FDA clearance by pointing out that the product used the company's material, made of Prolene, which had previously been OK'd by the FDA for hernia repair. In addition, the FDA had cleared it for an earlier Ethicon pelvic mesh, the Gynemesh PS, in 2002.

If a product uses the same mesh material, it must be a "substantially equivalent" device, yes?

No.

Prolift was a new kind of POP kit, created rapidly by J&J. Its structure was unique. The Prolift mesh had six arms and required special implant tools including a trocar (a sharp-pointed surgical instrument) and an insertion cannula (a small tube). The precut mesh consisted of a central implant with six straps or "arms"; four straps secured the anterior portion of the implant between the bladder and the vagina, and two others held the posterior portion in place between the rectum and the vagina. The straps extended into the hip, thigh, groin, and buttocks. They were intended to become fully integrated into the body.

And although it did use the same Gynemesh material as earlier Ethicon products, its size and implant technique were "completely different," according to one of Ethicon's doctors, Axel Arnaud.

Posterier Mesh Implant
The posterior mesh implant is constructed from GYNECARE GYNEMESH PS and is shaped for repair of posterior and/or apical vaginal vault defects. The implant has 2 straps that are secured in the bulbospongiosus ligament via a transvaginal approach. Alternatively, the 2 posterior straps may be put to reduce their length and secured in the sacrospinous ligament via a vaginal approach. The posterior straps have rounded ends (see Figure 1).

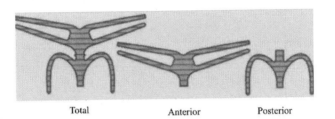

Total   Anterior   Posterior

Figure 1 - Mesh Implants (Total, Anterior, and Posterior)

GYNECARE PROLIFT Guide
The GYNECARE PROLIFT Guide is a single-patient-use instrument designed to create tissue paths to allow placement of the Total, Anterior, and Posterior mesh implants and to facilitate placement of the GYNECARE PROLIFT Cannula. Its length and curvature are specifically designed to create proper placement paths for all mesh implant straps. The GYNECARE PROLIFT Guide is suitable for use on both sides of the patient (see Figure 2).

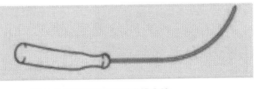

Figure 2 - GYNECARE PRODUCT Guide

Prolift inserted a larger volume of mesh into the pelvic space than did Gynemesh PS, according to court documents.

Concerns about Prolift started as it was being developed in the early 2000s. Ethicon had a team of doctors and researchers in France working on it. Already the group had questions about the amount of shrinkage possible using the relatively large mesh piece that would be part of the Prolift kit. For example, a 19–20 percent shrinkage could decrease the mesh size by up to 60 percent. One of those Ethicon consultants was Michel Cosson, a leading French urogynecologist and researcher. In July 2003, Dr. Cosson wrote to Ethicon, saying they had identified problems with the mesh material including erosion (exposure through the vaginal wall or into organs), contraction (scar tissue around the mesh pushes it together), and recurrence (the return of prolapse). Cosson said that if too much erosion occurred with the mesh, the team needed "to go back into the concept stage." J&J might even need to "delay launch."

Delay launch? Not likely.

In July 2003, Dr. Cosson wrote to Ethicon, saying they had identified problems with the mesh material including erosion (exposure through the vaginal wall or into organs), contraction (scar tissue around the mesh pushes it together), and recurrence (the return of prolapse). Cosson said that if too much erosion occurred with the mesh, the team needed "to go back into the concept stage." J&J might even need to "delay launch." Delay launch? Not likely.

SPINNING LIES

If you think you are about to read that J&J delayed the launch of Prolift to further test their mesh or the implant procedure's safety, put the book down now.

Ethicon didn't intend to lose any more time in the "speed to market" game with its rivals in the prolapse repair arena.

In January 2005, the scientific director of Gynecare Europe emailed the director who oversaw the marketing launch of Prolift worldwide, proposing to add a warning to the instructions for use (IFU). "Warning: Early clinical experience has shown that the use of mesh through a vaginal approach can occasionally/uncommonly lead to complications such as vaginal erosion and retraction, which can result in an anatomical distortion of the vaginal cavity that can interfere with sexual intercourse."

> In January 2005, the scientific director of Gynecare Europe emailed the director who oversaw the marketing launch of Prolift worldwide, proposing to add a warning to the instructions for use (IFU). "Warning: Early clinical experience has shown that the use of mesh through a vaginal approach can occasionally/ uncommonly lead to complications such as vaginal erosion and retraction, which can result in an anatomical distortion of the vaginal cavity that can interfere with sexual intercourse." The request bounced to Ethicon US. "We have already printed launch stock," wrote an employee there.

The risk increased if the patient had a hysterectomy. "This must be taken in consideration when the procedure is planned in a sexually active woman."

The request bounced to Ethicon US. "We have already printed launch stock," wrote an employee there. The warning was finally added three years later, after a nudge from the FDA.

But the French were right to worry about mesh extrusion upending one's sex life. In January 2008, a doctor who had met with one of Ethicon's executives wrote back about their discussion of dyspareunia linked to Prolift. "Actually, I am not using Prolift total vaginal mesh in sexually active patients under 60 unless they realize and acknowledge that there is a 5–10 percent risk of dyspareunia, as well as a 5 percent risk of erosion," he said.

In March 2005, Dr. Cosson, who was already a thorn in the side of another mesh maker, Mentor (ObTape), published an article with other members of Ethicon's French TVM group about a study of patients eight weeks after Prolift surgery.

Of 277 patients in the study, 34 women had experienced mesh exposure. After a month of treatment, 25 required surgery. Based on their data, the authors advised that "caution be exercised when carrying out this new surgical procedure."

They also suggested the company conduct "experimental studies and clinical trials . . . in order to reduce the level of exposure to less than 5 percent of cases."

Finally, Dr. Cosson asked a member of the R&D division back in the US to tell the higher-ups at Ethicon about the French team's concerns and their desire for a new, different mesh. Ethicon "just ignored us," said Dr. Cosson later in an interview for this book.

Perhaps that was because that same month Ethicon was busy preparing study submissions and presentations for the International Continence Society and the American Urogynecologic Society. They were going to introduce Prolift.

In emails from March 24, 2005, Ethicon executives discussed what risks to include or omit when talking about Prolift at upcoming doctors' meetings and how to present its data.

Regarding the revelation of some early complications in Prolift, one Ethicon email from Laura Angelini read, all in capitals, "I WOULD LIKE THAT WE SPIN IT MORE ON THE SAFETY ASPECT RATHER THAN COMPLICATIONS.

CAN WE INCLUDE THAT IN THE TITLE AS WELL?"

The "spin" suggestion continued: "I have attached a draft for our internal review only. Vince (Lucente) felt it was unethical to exclude dyspareunia data.

"I accept that we need to report the case of dyspareunia, because I agree that it would be unethical not to mention, since we know about it.

"However," the writer warned, "the way it is presented in the abstract is going to kill us."

Dyspareunia was one of the serious—and not that rare—side effects of many pelvic slings and POP kits. It is severe pain during sex sometimes caused by eroded plastic mesh poking through the vaginal wall. It can also scratch and hurt a penis, as mentioned.

> "I accept that we need to report the case of dyspareunia, because I agree that it would be unethical not to mention, since we know about it. "However," the writer warned, "the way it is presented in the abstract is going to kill us."

"We cannot really say anything on dyspareunia (and certainly cannot mention any percentage, if we have not really analyzed the data and asked the question)," the email continued.

"Maybe mention separately, and clearly say that this is one report . . ."

After more email exchanges, an Ethicon US executive responded to Angelini, "I will remove the dyspareunia, and if it comes up [during the conference], we can speak to it."

He added, "It is only self-reported as an adverse event and not solicited in a questionnaire . . ."

"To my knowledge, we will not have 'solicited' information [questionnaires] on dyspareunia [at the end of testing]. Therefore, there will be no scientific analysis specific to dyspareunia other than that which is reported as an adverse event."

This is how the professionals do it. Take an important adverse event and find a way to redefine its source. Find a way to limit its discussion.

It is only *ONE* report. And it's *self-reported*. Is that really enough to qualify as data? Is this enough to meet the criteria for scientific analysis?

In political polling, crafting a revisionist view of the data is called "massaging the message."

There was so much message massaging going on during the prolapse kit wave that companies should have put a spa in their marketing departments.

> "To my knowledge, we will not have 'solicited' information [questionnaires] on dyspareunia [at the end of testing]. Therefore, there will be no scientific analysis specific to dyspareunia other than that which is reported as an adverse event."

BAD PRODUCT, BIG PROFITS

US doctors started asking questions about problems with Prolift not long after it came to market in the spring of 2005. Implanting Prolift was more difficult than expected.

Dr. Vincent Lucente, an Ethicon preceptor and consultant, became the first doctor to implant the Prolift. He was very supportive of the device. When issues arose, Lucente, who had worked to fix the instructions for Ethicon's TVT-Secur, looked at ways to adapt the surgical insertion process for Prolift.

But it would not be easy to adjust the insertion procedure for Prolift with its six arms.

Menahem Neuman, the Flying Surgeon who had tracked the difficulties with Ethicon's TVT-Secur in Europe, had also seen problems with Prolift while he was training mesh doctors. "It is a difficult surgery; it can be dangerous," he said in an interview.

"I warned the company at the time that too many doctors did not have the skills for this. You could puncture a vessel. Many things could go wrong.

"And there was too much mesh in it," he added.

Dr. Neuman's worries were on target. Internal documents that surfaced later showed that the company was aware of how complex Prolift surgery was. "As of June 30, 2006, Ethicon knew, based on a document entitled 'Definition for MAJOR INVASIVE SURGERIES and the Ethicon Franchise Products Requiring Major Invasive Procedures for Implantation' that Prolift required major invasive surgery for its implantation," said a report using those documents.

Prolift wasn't becoming an overnight success. That fall, J&J's rival, American Medical Systems, mentioned Ethicon during its 2005 third-quarter earnings call. AMS told investors they welcomed news that with POP kits "the only other competitor in the market is Johnson & Johnson, and we are not seeing a lot from that."

"We are not in a position where we are having to worry about pricing; we are not in a position where there appears to be a lot of traction with their product from a competitive perspective, and so we are actually quite pleased with where we are," said an AMS chief.

AMS went on to announce that they had received such a positive analysis of their own Apogee and Perigee retrospective studies that they had decided to make the results public. Their data was "quite favorable" compared to other studies, "including the recent study published by Gynecare on their Prolift product," AMS said.

But PR efforts by Ethicon at various meetings with doctors at events for the American Urogynecologic Society and the American College of Obstetricians and Gynecologists over the next 18 months bolstered Prolift sales.

ANOTHER MESH CASUALTY

Ethicon was not alone in the POP kit debacle. Boston Scientific's Pinnacle prolapse kit and C. R. Bard's Avaulta were linked to a number of serious injuries. Avaulta had eight arms to Prolift's six. And Pinnacle implanted the most mesh of all in the vagina.

Removal of POP kit mesh is a marathon. Dr. Dionysios Veronikis took out an entire Prolift and put its picture on the Internet.

"I posted an entire Prolift—[it took] six hours [to remove]. I posted every bit of it up there, because I want the women of the world to know you can get help," said Dr. Veronikis. "People say, 'Veronikis, you don't need to do all that.'"

He disagrees. "Well, there is literature out there that talks about [the drawbacks of] partial removal, and how many follow-up surgeries the patients undergo.

"Six hours. Six hours," he adds.

The POP kits' explosion is reminiscent of one of the issues with the diet-drug combo fen-phen. When Redux, the "fen" part, was approved by the FDA, it was intended only for the morbidly obese. But company documents showed that Wyeth hoped to sell it to a much larger market.

Similarly, prolapse kits should have been used only for women who were in phase 3 or 4 of prolapse and incontinence, and they should have only been implanted by skilled surgeons. But such a narrow marketing base wasn't going to bring in the revenues that the mesh makers and their investors wanted.

Ethicon continued to push back against the FDA's insistence that it stop selling Prolift in 2005 until 2008, when the agency cleared the new Prolift + M, and the original Prolift, a kind of "grandfathering" of the older model. It wasn't until 2012 that Ethicon finally said it would withdraw Prolift from the market—for business reasons.

That was two years too late for one patient. Prolift implantation was, as Ethicon employees indicated in 2006, invasive surgery, with all its risks. In May 2010, an email was sent to key executives at the company.

The subject line was: "Patient deceased during a Prolift procedure."

"Dear colleagues,

I have been made aware yesterday that a patient died during a Prolift procedure. This is a very tragic event, and we feel sorry for this patient and her family," the doctor's email began. "The patient was aged 64 and had no comorbidities."

The surgeon had been trained on October 2007 in one of the Prolift centers in France. "Since then, the surgeon has been regularly using Prolift without problems," and was conducting some 30 Prolift procedures a year, the writer continued.

"What happened apparently is that the surgeons injured a big vessel and could not stop the bleeding. The patient received 20 units of blood, and eventually died on the table."

And still the dangers of mesh were kept secret.

SUZANNE EMMET'S STORY

Since we're talking about Prolift, let's bring the harsh truth of this dangerous device into the real world. We can talk about doctors, company executives, and those hiding behind the FDA, but the real impact of this tragedy is best told from a patient's point of view.

Suzanne thought the worst things that had happened to her after her Prolift mesh implant, besides the pain, were all the repair procedures—was it eight or nine?

Wait: maybe it was the loss of the warm physical relationship she enjoyed with her husband Mike.

Perhaps it was the burns from the medical sessions when silver nitrate was applied to places in her vagina to cauterize scar tissue around mesh that was poking out.

Or that terrible electric shock down her leg that neurologists administered every several months to control her endless bladder spasms.

Maybe it was how the urine would just run down her legs as she was talking with colleagues or her clients at the large insurance company where she was now senior vice president.

But none of that compared to what the lawsuit did to her—it opened her eyes. Our government protects us from dangerous medical products, and corporations don't sell anything they know could kill us, right? Titans of industry and world-class scientists—were they all so foolish that they put their secrets in memos and snarky emails?

Yes, the trial was the worst thing that happened to Suzanne. It destroyed what was left of her belief that the "system" works.

"Before this suit, I wouldn't have believed what they were all doing," says Suzanne.

"We go about our business as citizens of the US. We hear the FDA talked about in this reverential way—"the FDA has approved this."

"We're told the FDA has knowledge we don't have. We're told the company's scientists have knowledge and did due diligence. We're getting something that's safe. That's simply not true," she adds.

"I saw those emails. The arrogance. The nonchalance of those executives and the clinical people. They were joking about us and our husbands," she says.

Suzanne was like most young women growing up in the eastern half of Pennsylvania, and it was inevitable that she would take at least one summer vacation at the Jersey shore. She wanted to go to Wildwood.

The beach town was the subject of pop-rock songs. And the source of millions of teenage girls' memories—-walks on the sand holding hands with boys, the smell of Coppertone in the warm breeze on the beach clashing with the odor of cheesesteaks on the boardwalk.

That's where Suzanne met Mike Emmet. It was just about love at first sight.

Suzanne had more than marriage in her future. She'd already made plans for a career, getting a degree in 1983 from Franklin & Marshall College in Lancaster. She used that to propel herself into business.

Several years later, Suzanne helped found a new insurance company serving central Pennsylvania. Eventually, she became a senior vice president in charge of claims and compliance.

With what she learned while handling insurance problems, Suzanne became quite an expert on workers' compensation, including its gaps. She volunteered with Kids' Chance of America, a nationwide group that provides educational opportunities and scholarships to children of parents who die or are seriously injured on the job; she served a two-year term as its national president.

Suzanne and Mike had two children, a boy and a girl. She'd had difficult births with both; they were large infants.

In May 2007, Suzanne, bothered by increasing problems with stress incontinence, had surgery to alleviate prolapse. "It could be embarrassing at work, having to run to the restroom in the middle of something. It happened to me during presentations, at conventions . . ." She was implanted with Ethicon's POP kit Prolift and with its TVT-O incontinence sling. Her surgeon, Dr. Patricia Reddy, was experienced with the mesh implant, having been trained by a doctor who was one of the world's experts in mesh, the first doctor to implant a Prolift in the US, Dr. Vince Lucente.

Within a few months, Suzanne began experiencing a discharge with an unpleasant odor. There was discomfort; incontinence returned and got worse. And she began having pain during sex.

Suzanne returned to Dr. Reddy that fall. Reddy promptly contacted her mesh mentor, Dr. Lucente, at his hospital in Allentown just a couple of hours away.

Imagine you have trouble with your car and Dale Earnhardt Jr. offers to look at it for you. Or you can't make a decent jump shot on the court and Michael Jordan says he'll show you how.

Vincent Lucente was going to find out what was wrong with Suzanne Emmet and make it right.

Over the next six years Suzanne would visit Lucente a dozen times. "I think I had two revision surgeries with him at the hospital. I had several more procedures in his treatment center . . . And there were more extrusion 'trims' in his office," says Suzanne.

With the first revision surgery, "Dr. Lucente said the mesh had folded over, like it says in some of the documents, 'like a potato chip.' But there was a debate over how that happened. Dr. Lucente told me, 'I need to fix that.'"

However, she testified, Dr. Lucente did not tell her the source of her symptoms was the mesh implant itself, the Prolift. "In my mind, the way he described it, I was under the impression mesh was still there under my vaginal tissue. He would flatten it out," she says. "I didn't know it had actually eroded through vaginal tissue. That's not what he described to me.

"He said, 'This mesh is fine. This mesh is not the problem,'" Suzanne says. "'Suboptimal placement,' he told me."

Suzanne thought Dr. Lucente might be trying to say the Prolift and TVT-O that Dr. Reddy had implanted hadn't been inserted properly. But "that wasn't it," Suzanne said, citing documents.

After Lucente's revision surgery and procedures, Suzanne says things seemed OK for a couple of years, though there was continuing discomfort. But then, around 2011, all the earlier symptoms and new ones erupted in force. Vaginal bleeding, severe pain, and urinary tract infections that would not quit. Suzanne went back to Lucente.

During this time, in fact, from about 2000 to 2012, Lucente was playing a major role for Ethicon as one of its top key opinion leaders and a consultant, helping with developments and the use of their mesh products. Lucente was paid more than $1 million over that span by the company, according to court records.

Suzanne knew none of that. "Unbelievable," she says. The doctor who was treating her in relation to problems linked to Prolift mesh was also getting paid by the company that made it.

"Isn't that a conflict of interest?" Suzanne points out.

Lucente testified that he did not cite mesh as the cause of Suzanne's problems. He did begin telling patients that he was a consultant for Ethicon, Suzanne says.

Sometime in 2012, Suzanne saw an ad on TV about pelvic mesh problems and lawsuits. "I did research online and realized it had to be the mesh. Erosion."

"The next time I saw him, I asked, and he said there was nothing wrong with the mesh," Suzanne says.

Ethicon's defense attorneys "made a lot out of me being in insurance, what I knew about claims, statutes of limitations, evidence.

"But when I was in Dr. Lucente's office, I wasn't senior VP of claims, I was his patient—I was a woman who had a problem. I was sitting with a doctor whom I trusted completely. I had no reason not to trust him to help me."

Then learning about Lucente's long ties to Ethicon, "hearing what he knew . . . ," Suzanne says.

During her lengthy trial in Philadelphia that ended in January 2019, it was revealed that a lot of people knew something was wrong with Prolift and other mesh. Emails showed a company trying to control information about those problems with one of their most important products for female health.

In 2004, an Ethicon's clinical director, Dr. David Robinson, learned of two cases of women in Europe who couldn't void, or urinate, after getting Prolift.

In 2005, Robinson emailed Martin Weisberg who oversaw medical issues for the company. "I now have 4 cases of women who can't void" since their Prolift surgery. He'd heard of two more. In a couple instances, the problem resolved itself, but it took almost a year. "What was Ethicon doing about the matter?" Robinson asked.

"If this starts getting reported, it's going to scare the daylights out of docs."

The emails that really infuriated Suzanne involved post-Prolift intercourse. "Mike and I had a good relationship that way. Then I was in terrible pain. And then he got scratched really badly during sex one night." Mike wasn't the only husband or partner in the US getting injured by the mesh poking through his wife's vagina.

The problem had been identified years earlier. An internal J&J email in November 2005 said, "Hi—Have any ideas on Gynemesh erosion where only jagged edges are sticking out, not a whole sheet? I see 4 'whiskers' only, but it's a painful French tickler for the patient's husband."

Executive Martin Weisberg ended up apologizing for other emails that made fun of the man who had complained that making love to his wife, who had mesh, was like "screwing a wire brush." Responding to a note about the patient and the effects of her extrusion, Weisberg wrote, "I've never tried the wire brush thing, so I won't comment."

And of course, there were documents—more emails—about Ethicon's efforts to "spin" information, including data, for PR. In 2008, an Ethicon employee named Judith Gauld discussed her concerns with David Robinson. The exchange was read aloud during the trial.

"I do feel very strongly about the situation . . . I am really concerned that the lines between commercial and research . . . need to be clear-cut," she wrote. "And in this company, I am continually amazed and surprised at our need to push back. I understand the need to keep our relationship good with marketing and believe this is possible if we are trusted and respected to do our jobs. More importantly, for me, is that we are able to continue to work with the best uro-gyns in a research setting and that they see us behaving in an objective and scientifically robust manner."

Just above her signature, Ms. Gauld wrote, "Sorry about this, but I do need to say it, I will buy you a drink in London."

Robinson responded to her. "Well said, and I will take you up on the drink." He added, "Need to be careful."

Gauld wrote back, "I know what you're saying. My concern with (an Ethicon executive) is his closeness to EU marketing and his constant wish to 'spin' data, for example, TVT World interim (data), and therefore the loss of objectivity."

In 2009, one of the chiefs in the clinical division, Dr. Piet Hinoul, and Ethicon scientist Colin Urquhart, emailed each other about issues with the reporting of TVT mesh side effects. Writing about the company's "TVT World adverse event report," Dr. Hinoul said, "This is pretty awful. Obviously there are a lot of investigators who mistake an adverse outcome for an adverse event. Certain centres have a very high erosion rate it appears for continence tapes."

Hinoul's email continues, "I would not ask the investigators if they would change; tell them you will change unless they object."

Colin writes back, "Hi, Piet. Are you saying the red fields should be upgraded to 'possibly related' and the green fields are adverse outcomes?" He adds, "If so, the adverse outcomes cannot be amended, correct?"

Suzanne noted that she is a certified compliance and ethics professional—a CCEP—and one of her jobs over the past 21 years involves the compliance function. From that perspective, she says, "What I heard about the spinning of the data was shocking.

"The fact that if they had problems that were being reported, but that they were not soliciting, not asking about, they made the decision not to include those complaints in the database.

"It's like: we're not asking about it, so we don't have to track it—that's mind-blowing.

"The clinical director allowed himself to be swayed by pressure of the marketing people. That the (review) board made the decision there would be no clinical trials for Prolift.

"What got me was the total lack of accountability," she says. "If one person had stood up and said, 'This isn't right,' it would be a whole different world."

The jury found in favor of Suzanne. Ethicon is appealing the verdict and the generous amount awarded in punitive damages.

Suzanne said the jury awarded the punitive damages because it came across during the trial that Ethicon's culture is "poisoned."

Then, when Ethicon witnesses began talking about the company credo, she says, "That was a point when I couldn't sit in that courtroom. It made me physically ill. I had to get up and leave.

"Oh, there was one other time I left," she adds. "It was when they were going over the email about dyspareunia and women's pain during sex, and that one man suggested that sodomy was a good alternative.

"Right then, I got up and left to go to the restroom."

CHAPTER 10

THE IRREGULAR
REGULATORY PROCESS

"You may not market this device until you have
provided adequate information" on 16 potential deficiencies and received FDA approval.

"If you market the device without conforming
to these requirements, you will be in violation of
the Federal Food, Drug, and Cosmetic Act."

—Letter from the FDA to Johnson & Johnson, August 24, 2007, on Prolift

"Cut off a million clits in Africa, and
nobody hears a word. Cut one dick off, and
the whole fucking country stops."

—*New Yorker* story about the Lorena Bobbitt trial

Former scientists and doctors in the US Food and Drug Administration's
division that regulates medical devices, the Center for Devices and
Radiological Health (CDRH), don't mince words when describing the
agency where they worked.

"People say the medical device division is 'the Wild West.' Anything
goes. Anything can get approved. It's true."

"The press thinks that the FDA's drug division caves to industry a lot. But it's the medical device office that lets companies walk all over them. For *decades.*"

Those quotes came from former device scientists and reviewers who have extensive experience at the FDA and a stash of war stories about terrible products that made it to the US market despite some FDA officials' efforts to block them. Among the devices that triggered alarms with some FDA doctors were vaginal mesh implants, especially the POP kits for pelvic organ prolapse that started becoming popular in the mid-2000s.

> "We cleared dozens of slings and prolapse devices that were not tested for safety and efficacy. They got in because of that whole 'predicate' device scam. They're 'equivalent' to something else already on the market. It's a scam. I used to say it was a 'game,' but *game* is too innocuous—it's a scheme, a scam."

"We cleared dozens of slings and prolapse devices that were not tested for safety and efficacy. They got in because of that whole 'predicate' device scam. They're 'equivalent' to something else already on the market. It's a scam. I used to say it was a 'game,' but *game* is too innocuous—it's a scheme, a scam."

"The only people who benefit from it work for device makers or guys with stock in the companies," says one doctor with multiple degrees in medicine and science, who left the agency a few years ago. "When I tell my current colleagues tales of what went on at the FDA, they think I'm making it up. I say: 'Go look up this device or that device on the FDA site, and see how easy it was for a free pass.'

"Pelvic mesh? They tested that in rabbits. But not in their pelvises," he says. "They put a tiny slice of mesh in the rabbit under the skin on its back and its stays there, I don't know, days? If the rabbit doesn't drop dead or turn color, then the plastic is 'biocompatible.' Hey, quit laughing. I'm *not* kidding."

> "Pelvic mesh? They tested that in rabbits. But not in their pelvises," he says. "They put a tiny slice of mesh in the rabbit under the skin on its back and its stays there, I don't know, days? If the rabbit doesn't drop dead or turn color, then the plastic is 'biocompatible.' Hey, quit laughing. I'm *not* kidding."

And that's how experts explained the finer points of the science behind the 510(k) clearance process that allows an estimated 90–98 percent of medical devices to get fast-track clearance to the US market without actually testing the products in, say, humans.

One thing the device industry does pay to the government is user fees. The Medical Device User Fee Amendments (MDUFA) generate billions of dollars each year for the FDA (just as the Prescription Drug User Fee Act). Through MDUFA, device makers pay a fee to the agency in return for timely approval or clearance decisions for their devices. Agency reviewers are kept to an ironclad schedule demanded by the industry.

With this record of the Advanced Medical Technology Association's machinations and raw displays of power in Washington, is it any surprise that the Food and Drug Administration regulators, whose budget goes back to Congress every year, have used a light touch so often with medical device makers?

IGNORING THE CARNAGE
FOR A QUICK BUCK

In August 2007, the FDA sent a strongly worded letter—almost a threat—to the largest health-care products maker in America, Johnson & Johnson. The agency had caught J&J and its subsidiaries, Ethicon and Gynecare, *in flagrante delicto,* selling Prolift without regulatory approval. The company, as noted earlier, had been marketing the Prolift prolapse mesh kit since March 2005.

The agency said J&J/Ethicon could be breaking the law, violating one of the more serious parts of the Federal Food, Drug, and Cosmetic Act. By FDA standards, its missive read like a warning from *The Avengers* movies, demanding the return of Thor's hammer.

Unfortunately, the Prolift controversy became one of the best examples of the flaccid FDA inaction on medical devices.

That kind of warning letter could have sliced right into J&J's Women's Health division, panicking ob-gyns and urologists across the nation, sending them over to rivals Boston Scientific, C. R. Bard, and American Medical Systems. Any other company would probably be quaking with fear after such a demand from the government. But J&J wasn't *any other company.*

Johnson & Johnson had such a good relationship with federal regulators that it was shielded by the FDA, even as the agency fumed at them. The letter was not made public; as far as reporters or lawyers can tell, it was not posted with other "warning" letters to companies on the agency website. That meant no negative publicity for J&J investors, and no information slipping out to medical associations or physicians saying that Prolift was not ready for sale yet.

By this time in 2007, Prolift was already attracting complaints from patients and doctors about serious injuries during surgical implantation. Reports were filed complaining of severe side effects linked to the large amount of mesh used in the medical device and its somewhat awkward placement in patients. In fact, during the adverse event years that Prolift was being sold without official FDA clearance, there were 123 adverse event reports submitted to the FDA about the device.

But covered by a blanket of silence, Johnson & Johnson was able to dig in during the fall of 2007 for an extended nine-month fight with the FDA—during which time J&J continued to sell Prolift.

J&J'S FREE PASS

You see, there was more at stake. Ethicon was planning to launch its "new and improved" version of Prolift in 2008 that would be called Prolift + M. The company was already preparing documentation to apply for a fast-track clearance under the 510(k) loophole.

So, back at HQ in New Brunswick, it was business as usual. J&J's annual report for 2007 touted an 11.8 percent growth for Ethicon franchise revenues hitting $3.6 billion. That number was partly due to "solid growth" in the Women's Health division and "the mesh product lines."

Behind the scenes, J&J's attorneys and regulatory experts were pushing back against requests from FDA reviewers for "adequate information"—more data—on the safety of the original Prolift. The company insisted it had not violated the law, writing that its Prolift was predicated on its Gynemesh, cleared in 2002. J&J's application for Prolift + M said the original Prolift was an "insignificant change" from Gynemesh, according to stories in Bloomberg News and NJ.com.

According to a former FDA medical device official, device reviewers dealing with Prolift mesh didn't get much support from superiors at the medical device division.

Johnson & Johnson could have been fined millions of dollars, faced an injunction against the company or high-level executives, perhaps had one or more products waiting for review put on hold, or had its prolapse meshes seized by the government, according to a professor at Georgetown University Law Center.

If the tussle had been made public, it could have had "negative consequences" for the company, showing that J&J had been desperate in 2005 to get its first POP kit on the market, he said. "This was a serious legal issue, basic to the working of the system of safety checks involving our health-care products."

In the end, nothing happened. The FDA decided that J&J had acted in good faith because they believed they had met all the requirements for marketing Prolift and because it was covered by Gynemesh PS. The agency cleared Prolift + M in May 2008, using 510(k), and it retroactively cleared the original Prolift as well.

The wild Prolift story was not revealed until 2012, by Bloomberg News, in an article headlined "J&J ignored order to stop selling mesh." Plaintiffs' lawyers who were suing Ethicon over alleged Prolift-linked injuries had found the 2007–8 FDA/J&J correspondence during pre-trial discovery.

After Bloomberg reported on the Prolift outrage, J&J defended itself, saying the FDA's tough August 2007 letter had been "taken out of context." The letter, a company spokesperson told Bloomberg, was "only one part of an extended dialogue in 2007–8." J&J's "actions were responsible, appropriate and consistent with FDA regulations."

WHAT DO KNEES AND VAGINAS HAVE IN COMMON? ASK THE FDA

In the waning days of 2008, the Food and Drug Administration approved a new medical device for knee surgery. It was designed to help repair a torn meniscus, which orthopedic surgeons across America called the "Holy Grail of Knee Surgery." The Menaflex knee implant was intended to hold meniscus pieces together while tissue grew around it, ultimately providing stability for walking, jogging, and exercising.

Menaflex was approved through the 510(k) process. In this case, the makers of Menaflex—in New Jersey—said in FDA filings that the Menaflex knee repair implant was similar to a product that had been around for more than two decades: hernia mesh. (Sound familiar?)

Top device scientists and reviewers at the FDA were furious. They strenuously opposed its fast-track clearance. They were overruled by the then chief of the Center for Devices and Radiological Health Dan Schultz.

A couple FDA scientists leaked the internal documents on Menaflex to a congressional committee that oversees the FDA. The documents included tantalizing emails showing that members of New Jersey's delegation in the Capitol had prodded the FDA and its commissioner repeatedly to approve Menaflex.

Thanks to leaky congressional aides, the story about this debacle broke in the *Wall Street Journal* in March 2009.

There was a backlash among politicians not from New Jersey. And the incoming FDA commissioner, just appointed by the new president Barack Obama, launched a massive investigation. The emails involving members of Congress and the Senate and the outgoing FDA commissioner Andrew von Eschenbach got all the publicity.

But the most interesting documents—those involving science and public health policy—were those in which FDA device reviewers and members of the FDA's Medical Devices Advisory Committee kept complaining about Menaflex's "predicate" device.

It was hernia mesh. Yes, *that* hernia mesh. Reviewers complained that hernia mesh was originally intended for implant in a relatively large, flat area like the abdomen. Hernia mesh was never intended to be put into a joint, particularly a weight-bearing joint, particularly the knee.

If you're one of the two million women who have had vaginal mesh implants, you may think that this story has been put on repeat. Yes, hernia mesh is the duct tape of medical devices—apparently, there is no medical problem that cannot be solved by hernia mesh.

The fallout from Menaflex gave great hope to FDA scientists who told Congress that medical device approvals and clearances were out of control at the agency. As one scientist said, the device makers' lobbyists had been running the show. The agency released an unprecedented report criticizing former commissioner von Eschenbach and Dr. Schultz of the device division. It slammed the interference of lobbying and politics in the medical decision-making. The chief of the FDA device division announced his resignation and a couple other FDA officials left their jobs over the next several months.

Then the FDA announced that it was going to review the entire 510(k) process with an eye to reforming it to prevent abuse of "predicate" references. The agency wanted to curtail manufacturers looking for shortcuts to get their devices on the lucrative US market. The US Institute of Medicine (now part of the National Academy of Sciences) was tasked with producing an independent review of the 510(k) process, and committees all over the Capitol began investigations into the FDA's device sector.

DEVICE MAKERS DON'T LIKE TO LOSE

But the Food and Drug Administration could never outplay the medical device industry, says a former device official. Device makers wield more power than drug companies in the FDA and in the Capitol. "They don't take no for an answer," said several former and current FDA employees.

> Device makers wield more power than drug companies in the FDA and in the Capitol. "They don't take no for an answer," said several former and current FDA employees.

AdvaMed mobilized quickly when the FDA report on the Menaflex mess was released to the public. The lines between Republicans and Democrats began to blur. A former Washington lobbyist for several large device distributors reminded reporters about the geographic diversity of the device industry.

"Some of the major manufacturers are in states that you think of as Democratic," like Minnesota and Massachusetts, he said. That nullified a number of Democrats in the House and Senate. Republicans had no incentive to attack device makers who were always reliable donors to politicians they could rely on.

"We never knew what hit us," said a leading official at the FDA about the effort to bring the 510(k) loophole under control.

AdvaMed powered through agency hearings, and device maker representatives and additional lobbyists cluttered the corridors on Capitol Hill. Between 2009 and 2011, the device industry spent some $86 million on lobbying, according to the Union of Concerned Scientists. They also spent $24 million in 2008 on political donations according to OpenSecrets.org.

> Between 2009 and 2011, the device industry spent some $86 million on lobbying, according to the Union of Concerned Scientists. They also spent $24 million in 2008 on political donations according to OpenSecrets.org.

In 2011, Republicans took control of the House of Representatives and any move to reform the 510(k) process at the FDA died (despite hand-wringing by a few senators and outrage from major consumer advocates like Public Citizen). In fact, the FDA barely survived efforts by medical device makers to get congressional legislation passed that would enlarge the 510(k) loophole, loosen more FDA regulations on device makers, and basically lock scientific integrity in the broom closet.

"One proposal would change the FDA's mission to include job creation, reducing the scrutiny the agency could give to medical devices by compelling the agency to consider every 'least burdensome' alternative to improving device safety. Another would erode the FDA's standard of 'substantial evidence' when reviewing drugs and devices," warned the Union of Concerned Scientists.

While the Menaflex scandal had been playing out, the makers of vaginal mesh were holding their breath. They had spent a dozen years staying a step ahead of US regulators, using 510(k). That hernia mesh predicate was pretty important to them because literally dozens of vaginal implants for incontinence and prolapse were based on Ye Olde Hernia Meshe.

You could hear their collective sigh of relief across the Potomac.

By the end of July 2011, when the Institute of Medicine (IOM) released its report calling for a quick end to the 510(k) program, AdvaMed had already won. The FDA responded meekly to the report it had requested from IOM, saying the agency "believes that the 510(k) process should not be eliminated." But, it said, the FDA is "open to additional proposals and approaches for continued improvement of our device review programs."

> Yes, how exactly does a device maker obtain both a patent for a "new" device, while also begging for a "substantially equivalent" label, thus avoiding clinical testing and studies?

Too bad. The 510(k) isn't just a regulatory loophole; it's a conundrum of metaphysical proportions.

In a riveting book on medical implants called *The Danger Within Us*, author Jeanne Lenzer writes, "The double-edged sword of being 'different,' while simultaneously claiming 'substantial equivalence' has created a logical loophole exploited by industry, which the IOM concluded can't be repaired."

Yes, how exactly does a device maker obtain both a patent for a "new" device, while also begging for a "substantially equivalent" label, thus avoiding clinical testing and studies?

Lenzer found a clue in a revelatory talk given a few years ago by an ex-official at CDRH.

Donna-Bea Tillman, the former director of the Office of Device Evaluation, who left the FDA in 2010, spoke about the ways device entrepreneurs must navigate the "nuances" of the 510(k) pathway.

"The 510(k) is the pathway that most people who are developing new medical devices are likely to run into, and it is the pathway that requires you to identify a predicate device, which is a legally marketed device, to show that your new device is substantially equivalent. So that's what you need to do," she said.

"And it's kind of interesting, because what I find is that a lot of my clients say, 'Oh, my device is novel and it's new, and there's nothing else like it out there.'"

But, Tillman said, "That is absolutely *not* what you want to tell the FDA, because you want to be able to say to the FDA, 'Well, yes, even though I may have some new features or a slightly different technology, it's substantially equivalent to what's already out there.'

"*That's* what enables you to go through this 510(k) pathway, which is a lot less costly and expensive and burdensome than going down the PMA [premarket approval] pathway."

It saves the companies a lot. What it saves patients is a different question.

BACK AT THE RANCH

Dr. Diana Zuckerman and her think tank, which was begun in 1999, have been on the "mesh watch" for more than a decade. She is a well-known expert in the nation's capital on the safety and effectiveness of medical products, especially devices used in women's health care.

As a congressional investigator in 1990, her work exposed the fact that breast implants had never been studied in women—which probably sounds familiar to those following the vaginal mesh disaster.

That news prompted extensive media coverage of the breast implants. They were sold for 20-some years, often leaking into women's bodies and could lead to systemic medical problems. Medical researchers, with the support of a major breast implant maker, called Dr. Zuckerman's warnings about breast implants "junk science."

But several years ago, the FDA and medical researchers began warning about an unusual cancer—*not* breast cancer, but a cancer of the immune system that developed just outside breast implants—possibly linked to silicone or saline-filled implants. Since then, it has been established that anaplastic large cell lymphoma can be caused by breast implants, and there is growing recognition that many women with breast implants experience autoimmune reactions that mimic conditions like lupus and rheumatoid arthritis. Diana Zuckerman could have said, "I told you so," but good manners stopped her.

After her center was up and running, Zuckerman said, "One of the first requests we got from the public was 'What can you do about mesh?' The only thing I knew was that it served as the predicate for TMJ (teeth grinding prevention) implants," said Dr. Zuckerman. Vaginal mesh and your jaw—why not?

Using her experience as a congressional investigator, Zuckerman did a briefing on Capitol Hill. She coordinated some of her mesh work with a small patient advocacy group. The group had arranged for a meeting with representatives from AUGS, the American Urogynecologic Society. The head of the advocacy group hoped that the meeting with AUGS would lead to changes in the growing use of vaginal mesh by doctors.

"That did not go as planned," says Zuckerman. "The AUGS people were completely defensive, expressed no support for patients who had been harmed," says Zuckerman. The AUGS message was "there are 'bad' doctors out there, though very few do a bad job. And it's certainly not our doctors at AUGS doing bad jobs. And the problem is definitely *not* the mesh . . ."

At an AUGS meeting later on, which Zuckerman attended, the president of AUGS gave a surprising keynote address, "talking about what a disgrace the 510(k) process was," Zuckerman says. The president said 510(k) put doctors in an unfair position, thinking that products were tested in clinical trials using humans. Zuckerman got in touch with the president afterward, and he told her the response to his speech was not favorable. He had hoped to "accomplish something," but in the end was ostracized, she said.

Zuckerman, who has been part of FDA working groups, has developed a good relationship with veteran regulators. She is familiar with some of the behind-the-scenes struggles over vaginal mesh.

There was little control by the FDA over mesh implants in the 1997–2007 era. But by 2008, the agency's dreadful adverse events reporting system for medical devices, called MAUDE, actually showed a rising number of incoming complaints about incontinence slings and, more worrisome, prolapse mesh kits.

> Doctors are not required to file reports to the FDA if a patient has a bad reaction to a drug or a medical device such as an implant. Though device/drug makers and hospitals must report serious problems, reporting is voluntary for America's tens of thousands of doctors, and the paperwork is frankly cumbersome. No wonder only about 10 percent of adverse events in the US are formally reported.

Because any "regulation" is anathema to health-care industry professionals, doctors are not required to file reports to the FDA if a patient has a bad reaction to a drug or a medical device such as an implant. Though device/drug makers and hospitals must report serious problems, reporting is voluntary for America's tens of thousands of doctors, and the paperwork is frankly cumbersome. No wonder only about 10 percent of adverse events in the US are formally reported.

But even with minimal useful data coming into the FDA, MAUDE revealed a trend in vaginal mesh reports. "This time, the FDA did not ignore it," says Zuckerman.

In October 2008, the FDA issued a safety communication about vaginal mesh implants to doctors. "This is to alert you to complications associated with transvaginal placement of surgical mesh" for incontinence and prolapse. "Although rare, these complications can have serious consequences."

It continued. Over the past three years, the FDA has received more than 1,000 reports from nine surgical mesh manufacturers of complications linked to POP and SUI vaginal meshes.

The 2008 notice is hardly alarming; the statement was released only after discussions with the companies that stressed the inclusion of "although rare." "But it was a start," says Dr. Zuckerman.

And while this was a step in the right direction, this passive notice was received much like junk mail that carelessly gets tossed on the already-high stacks of paperwork.

"December 19, 2009, was the worst day of my life," states Nancy Gretzinger, from Phoenix, Arizona. "I was assured by the surgeon implanting the two meshes for my condition was a simple procedure and she had completed many with no problems. She mentioned nothing of the FDA 2008 notification."

Obviously, Gretzinger was not alone. Most doctors never mentioned that the implant is permanent nor that additional surgeries may be required. It must have also slipped the surgeon's mind that there's a potential for serious complications that could affect quality of life. "Unfortunately, after eight surgeries, multiple procedures and drugs, my bladder neck was removed and a suprapubic catheter was inserted into my bladder. Other effects are evolving—decreased immunity, resistance to antibiotics, and other risks including possible bladder cancer."

So while the FDA notifications were being ignored during the frenzy over the knee mesh Menaflex, Zuckerman carefully tracked different excuses offered by the device industry to preempt a demand for real clinical trials and studies in humans—of course, many of them involved vaginal mesh.

"Sometimes I wonder if I'm just running in circles," she says. "If it's an *implant*, you test it before you put it *in*. And before you sell it."

Zuckerman has a message to the people in the 510(k) world of "basically unregulated devices":

"If you don't want to be in a business that requires clinical trials,
if you don't want to be regulated,
if you're not willing to test to see if your product is safe and effective,

if you want to make something that people's lives *don't* depend on, I say make shirts or buttons."

FDA JOINS THE PARTY

Just when the ruckus over 510(k) "reform" was dying down, the FDA released a surprising report that said there had been a fivefold increase in the number of deaths and injuries of malfunctions related to prolapse mesh implants. Unlike its 2008 safety alert, the July 2011 FDA paper said that serious side effects were "NOT rare." It also said that there was little data, if any, showing that vaginal mesh implants for prolapse were any more effective than traditional abdominal surgical procedures.

According to a former FDA official who handled some of the furor raised by doctors and patients, politicians and the press, the agency was strongly opposed by industry and industry-funded medical associations, who objected to the phrase "NOT rare," among other things. "It was a real struggle to get the paper approved and released to the public," she said in interviews. There was much pressure on the administration from the device industry, its lobbyists, and lawmakers on Capitol Hill.

That September, the FDA held a two-day advisory committee meeting on ob-gyn and urogynecological products.

AdvaMed went into "warp drive," said a former high-ranking FDA official. The device makers' lobbyists were not focused on the impact of potential new FDA actions on vaginal mesh. There was a more important issue in play that they could not afford to lose: the prized 510(k) clearance process.

During the meeting, some medical experts and doctors on the committee openly supported the idea of clinical trials or at least better studies involving humans before further vaginal mesh implant approvals. After all, there were another 1,500 "complications" reported in POP kit prolapse surgeries and a 36 percent increase in problems in stress urinary incontinence implants.

A number of members were also prepared to recommend reclassifying vaginal mesh—mostly the prolapse kit mesh—from Class II (medium risk) to Class III (high risk). A device in the Class III category needs to go through the premarket approval process, not the 510(k), and that involves a clinical study.

Panel member Dr. Cheryl Igesia of Washington, DC, had been part of an important study of vaginal mesh that was abruptly shut down in 2009 because of too many instances of mesh erosion. In discussing one of the issues before the committee, she said, "Unfortunately, through the 510(k) process, we've had some bad products that have been cleared, such as the ObTape . . . and the IVS Tunneller." Iglesia continued, "My fear is, in some sense, that I don't want that type of thing to ever hit the market again because that's what leads to the long-term risks."

As the meeting pushed forward, the topic of the problem-prone mini-slings came up. The FDA wanted the committee to decide if there was enough evidence on mini-slings' safety and effectiveness. Since there had been no real studies on the mini-slings before they were marketed, as several panel members mentioned, that question almost answered itself.

Dr. Iglesia laid out her objections to those devices. "There is not adequate safety and effectiveness data for the mini-slings." She commented on a recent trial presented to the International Urogynecological Association comparing the full-length TVT mesh to the mini-TVT-Secur sling looking at one-year data. The two devices had similar results in the incontinence severity index, complications, and pain scores. "But the mini-sling, when it failed, it failed worse," she said. "So definitely not ready for prime time," she added.

One of the witnesses invited by the FDA to testify was Dr. Tom Margolis, who was not shy when expressing his concerns about vaginal mesh. "The implantation of contaminated synthetic mesh through the vagina defies basic surgical tenets because, by definition, it is not performed in a sterile manner. So-called mesh erosion is really 'mesh infection with chronic wound breakdown.'

"Time does not permit me to expound upon the plethora of other complications associated with transvaginal mesh," Margolis said, proceeding to expound. He listed "damage to bowel, bladder and blood vessels, vaginal scarring, dyspareunia, need for multiple repairs, and destroyed personal lives."

Device makers and their lobby had created an ad hoc group for the meeting, the Transvaginal Mesh Industry Working Group. Members included AdvaMed, American Medical Systems, Bard Medical, Boston Scientific, Ethicon's Women's Health & Urology, with assistance from Covidien, W. L. Gore, and Coloplast.

Speaking for them at the Advisory Committee meeting was Ethicon's medical director for devices, Piet Hinoul, a well-known physician who had watched various meshes succeed and fail in Europe and the US.

> As Slater puts it, once a witness has sworn that the side effects are already "known" to some degree, the witness—and the company where the witness works—can't distance themselves from the side effects. Either the side effects were possible, because the product was approved through its equivalent "predicate," or they were unexpected—which meant the device should not have been allowed to use a 510(k) pass. It was not "equivalent" after all.

"Hinoul really had one job: protect the 510(k)," says plaintiffs' lawyer Adam Slater of New Jersey. Slater's opinion is that in order to show the FDA that the vaginal mesh lines were legitimately based on early predicate devices, the industry—Dr. Hinoul—had to make the case that none of the side effects that were known to be crippling women permanently in countries around the world were a surprise.

A product that is "substantially equivalent" to a predicate device "cannot have any surprises," he explains. And so, Dr. Hinoul and others working with the AdvaMed-industry team were in the position of defending terrible injuries as side effects that were known in advance to be "possible." Very rare, but "possible."

The vaginal mesh devices' side effects had been placed on the different products IFUs—instructions for use, Hinoul said.

Slater and his colleagues at the Mazie Slater firm read the transcripts of the two-day hearing several times. When the lawsuits started piling up, Slater's team would have what they needed to at least back the company Ethicon, Pinoul's employer, into a corner.

As Slater puts it, once a witness has sworn that the side effects are already "known" to some degree, the witness—and the company where the witness works—can't distance themselves from the side effects. Either the side effects were possible, because the product was approved through its equivalent "predicate," or they were unexpected—which meant the device should not have been allowed to use a 510(k) pass. It was not "equivalent" after all.

Some plaintiffs' lawyers would get to take Dr. Hinoul's deposition for the federal mass tort and New Jersey tort cases that were slowly coming together, and Adam Slater hoped he knew who that would be.

FDA FINALLY CLASSIFIES MESH AS "HIGH RISK"

Just 48 hours after New Year's Day 2012, the FDA announced it would request new "522" studies from the makers of vaginal mesh for incontinence "mini-slings" and for prolapse kits including Ethicon, Boston Scientific, and American Medical Systems. The FDA's notice signaled that it was considering reclassifying both the difficult "mini-sling" and the POP kits to the Class III risk category.

Manufacturers began to announce their planned voluntary withdrawal of prolapse kits and some other meshes from the market for "business reasons," which included avoiding the cost of and any negative results from such studies.

Among Ethicon's list of withdrawals over the next year were the Prolift, the Prolift + M, and the TVT-Secur System mini-sling. The company also said it was restricting the use of its Gynemesh nonabsorbable Prolene Soft mesh.

> By the end of 2012, the largest mass tort in the US since the asbestos cases had come together. The FDA was about to find out how much they did not know about vaginal mesh.

Was no one going to stand up for mesh?

Yes: the medical associations for urogynecologists (AUGS) and for ob-gyns (ACOG). They issued statements reasserting their support for vaginal mesh slings and the prolapse kits. The organizations would hang on until the end . . . or longer if necessary.

By the end of 2012, the largest mass tort in the US since the asbestos cases had come together. The FDA was about to find out how much they did not know about vaginal mesh.

Nonetheless, it took until 2016 for the FDA to officially categorize vaginal prolapse mesh as a Class III risk.

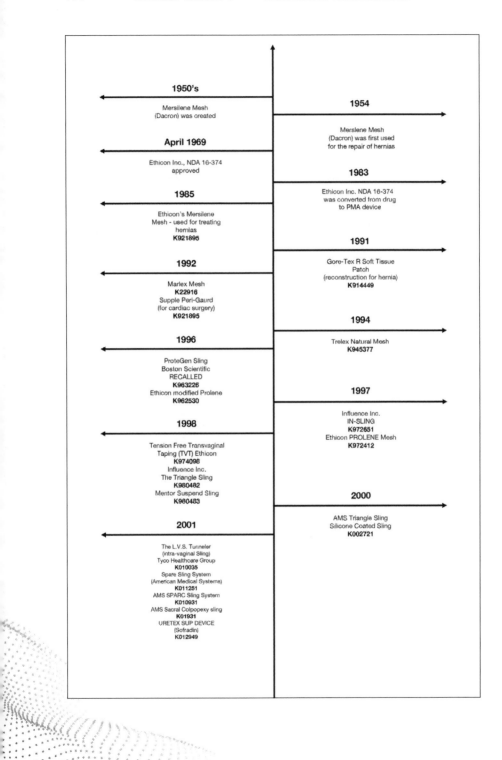

1950's

Mersilene Mesh
(Dacron) was created

1954

Mersilene Mesh
(Dacron) was first used
for the repair of hernias

April 1969

Ethicon Inc., NDA 16-374
approved

1983

Ethicon Inc. NDA 16-374
was converted from drug
to PMA device

1985

Ethicon's Mersilene
Mesh - used for treating
hernias
K921895

1991

Gore-Tex R Soft Tissue
Patch
(reconstruction for hernia)
K914449

1992

Marlex Mesh
K22916
Supple Peri-Gaurd
(for cardiac surgery)
K921895

1994

Trelex Natural Mesh
K945377

1996

ProteGen Sling
Boston Scientific
RECALLED
K963226
Ethicon modified Prolene
K962530

1997

Influence Inc.
IN-SLING
K972651
Ethicon PROLENE Mesh
K972412

1998

Tension Free Transvaginal
Taping (TVT) Ethicon
K974098
Influence Inc.
The Triangle Sling
K980482
Mentor Suspend Sling
K980483

2000

AMS Triangle Sling
Silicone Coated Sling
K002721

2001

The L.V.S. Tunneler
(intra-vaginal Sling)
Tyco Healthcare Group
K010035
Spare Sling System
(American Medical Systems)
K011251
AMS SPARC Sling System
K010931
AMS Sacral Colpopexy sling
K01931
URETEX SUP DEVICE
(Sofradin)
K012949

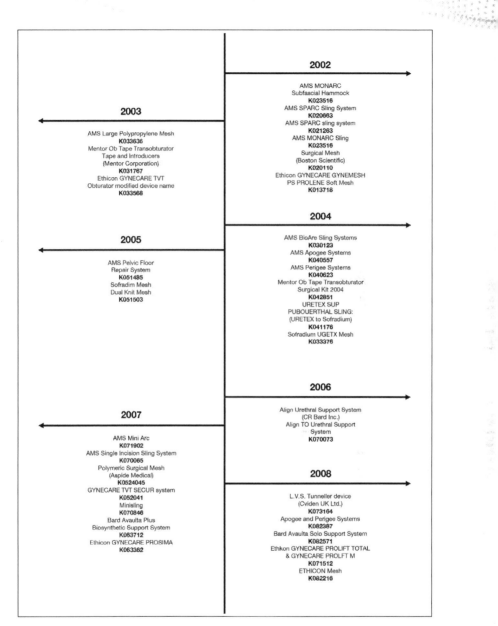

2002

AMS MONARC
Subfascial Hammock
K023516
AMS SPARC Sling System
K020663
AMS SPARC sling system
K021263
AMS MONARC Sling
K023516
Surgical Mesh
(Boston Scientific)
K020110
Ethicon GYNECARE GYNEMESH
PS PROLENE Soft Mesh
K013718

2003

AMS Large Polypropylene Mesh
K033636
Mentor Ob Tape Transobturator
Tape and Introducers
(Mentor Corporation)
K031767
Ethicon GYNECARE TVT
Obturator modified device name
K033568

2004

AMS BioAre Sling Systems
K030123
AMS Apogee Systems
K040557
AMS Perigee Systems
K040623
Mentor Ob Tape Transobturator
Surgical Kit 2004
K042851
URETEX SUP
PUBOUERTHAL SLING:
(URETEX to Sofradium)
K041176
Sofradium UGETX Mesh
K033376

2005

AMS Pelvic Floor
Repair System
K051485
Sofradim Mesh
Dual Knit Mesh
K051503

2006

Align Urethral Support System
(CR Bard Inc.)
Align TO Urethral Support
System
K070073

2007

AMS Mini Arc
K071902
AMS Single Incision Sling System
K070065
Polymeric Surgical Mesh
(Aspide Medical)
K0524045
GYNECARE TVT SECUR system
K052041
Minisling
K070846
Bard Avaulta Plus
Biosynthetic Support System
K063712
Ethicon GYNECARE PROSIMA
K063362

2008

L.V.S. Tunneller device
(Cviden UK Ltd.)
K073164
Apogee and Perigee Systems
K082387
Bard Avaulta Solo Support System
K082571
Ethkon GYNECARE PROLIFT TOTAL
& GYNECARE PROLFT M
K071512
ETHICON Mesh
K082216

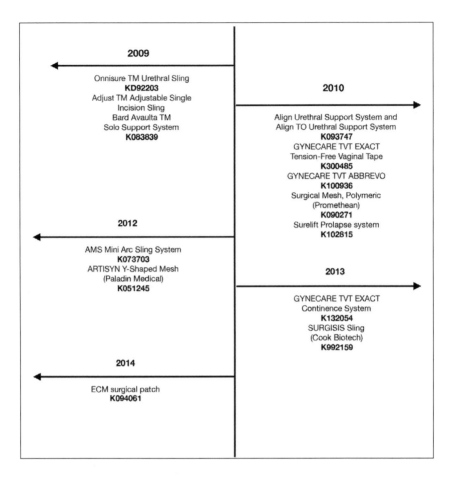

2009

Onnisure TM Urethral Sling
KD92203
Adjust TM Adjustable Single
Incision Sling
Bard Avaulta TM
Solo Support System
K083839

2010

Align Urethral Support System and
Align TO Urethral Support System
K093747
GYNECARE TVT EXACT
Tension-Free Vaginal Tape
K300485
GYNECARE TVT ABBREVO
K100936
Surgical Mesh, Polymeric
(Promethean)
K090271
Surelift Prolapse system
K102815

2012

AMS Mini Arc Sling System
K073703
ARTISYN Y-Shaped Mesh
(Paladin Medical)
K051245

2013

GYNECARE TVT EXACT
Continence System
K132054
SURGISIS Sling
(Cook Biotech)
K992159

2014

ECM surgical patch
K094061

CHAPTER 11

DEMIGODS

What's the difference between God and doctors?
God doesn't think he's a doctor.

I asked myself the question: WHY? I said: "Look,
we have created a monster! What could happen
to these women as this young population ages?"

—Dr. Shlomo Raz

What role did the doctors play in this gigantic mesh debacle? Did they know what they were doing and the devastation they were causing?

In other product liability disasters, doctors got a pass. The reason usually given for that is physicians and surgeons weren't told the truth about the drugs or the devices they were prescribing for patients. Companies kept "doctors in the dark."

But doctors haven't been passive in the vaginal mesh fiasco. They've been a big part of the problem. If they are still in the dark, it's because they don't want to turn on the lights.

Even now, most doctors in urogynecology won't even admit there *is* a major problem. Ruined vaginas, ruined lives? "Those are such *rare* events with mesh implants," they say. "Discomfort, dyspareunia, and Depend? Those aren't *severe* side effects," the doctors say.

All those pitches by device makers' sales reps about the "easy money" in mesh, the Lamborghinis, the quickie surgeries that would allow a doctor to make tee time at the golf course—they *worked.*

All those pitches by device makers' sales reps about the "easy money" in mesh, the Lamborghinis, the quickie surgeries that would allow a doctor to make tee time at the golf course—they *worked.* By 2006, physicians were doing 100,000 mesh implants a year in the US. The incontinence sling and the prolapse kits, they were juggernauts that could not be stopped.

And many doctors made a fortune "advising" corporations, training wanna-be surgeons in the intricacies of difficult vaginal mesh implants, and filing patents for new devices they helped design, which resulted in lucrative royalty streams directly into their bank accounts.

By 2006, physicians were doing 100,000 mesh implants a year in the US. The incontinence sling and the prolapse kits, they were juggernauts that could not be stopped. The evidence is laid out in thousands of internal company documents, emails, and financial analyses involving individual doctors, mesh "mills," and the medical associations that represent them. Together they show that a segment of the medical community was so heavily invested in the success of vaginal mesh implants that it ignored or suppressed mounting evidence of dangers and permanent damage to women.

Doctors' failure to protect their patients is one of the most troubling chapters in the saga of the pelvic mesh craze.

THE EXPERIMENTAL EXPERIENCE

One shameful example that demonstrates the financial dependence of the gynecological community on mesh maker corporations involved a major battle over a minor edit in a medical publication.

In 2007, one word in a Practice Bulletin issued by the American College of Obstetricians and Gynecologists about prolapse implants caused an explosion in the mesh business.

"Given the limited data and frequent changes in marketed products (particularly with regard to type of mesh material itself, which is most closely associated with several of the postoperative risks, especially mesh erosion), the procedures should be considered *experimental*, and patients should consent to surgery with that understanding."

A mere seven months later, a revised Practice Bulletin was released. In the new guidance, the word "experimental" had been surgically excised, like a tumor.

ACOG's controversial Practice Bulletin was published in February that year. Doctors, their medical associations, and mesh makers were apoplectic and decided to "fix the problem," according to a physician involved. A fight ensued behind the scenes involving the author, prestigious doctors in ACOG and AUGS, and of course, the companies.

A mere seven months later, a revised Practice Bulletin was released. In the new guidance, the word "experimental" had been surgically excised, like a tumor.

The seven-month turnaround was astounding, according to doctors who deal frequently with ACOG. Normally, said one, the society's Practice Bulletins are only reviewed every 18 months or longer.

ACOG's message was that "experimental" was "ambiguous" and confusing to the hundreds of doctors who had been doing mesh implants. However, the author of the bulletin, Dr. Anne Weber, wasn't fooled by the medical groups' excuses.

Anne Weber was not some intern new to medical studies. Weber is a urogynecologist—that ob-gyn specialty practice involving a year or more of extra training in surgery. She had been named the first director of the National Institutes of Health's innovative program on pelvic prolapse disorder. Weber had been immersed in issues and studies involving vaginal mesh implants for years.

> "Experimental" procedures, you see, aren't usually covered by third-party insurance. Without insurance payments, far fewer women would be opting for mesh prolapse surgeries and those paint-by-numbers POP kits.

She knew the real problem with her sentence was that vaginal mesh surgeries were still in the "experimental phase." The furor she created was not about etymology. It was about *money.*

"Experimental" procedures, you see, aren't usually covered by third-party insurance. Without insurance payments, far fewer women would be opting for mesh prolapse surgeries and those paint-by-numbers POP kits.

Dr. Weber "vehemently opposed" ACOG's changes, according to a later story on NPR station WBUR. In her interview with NPR, she went straight to the financial issue. "I think ACOG was choosing to protect its clinicians' insurance incomes over patients' well-being," she said.

She wasn't alone in that perception.

Dr. Lewis Wall, an influential urogynecologist at Washington University in St. Louis, complained to colleagues and others about ACOG's changes. He castigated ACOG later in a medical journal editorial coauthored with Douglas Brown. This critical article's title pretty much covered its conclusions: "Commercial Pressures and Professional

Ethics: Troubling Revisions to the Recent ACOG Practice Bulletins on Surgery for Pelvic Organ Prolapse."

By cutting "experimental" and altering the bulletin's text, Wall and Brown wrote, "The ACOG Committee on Practice Bulletins shifts the responsibility for using these procedures from the surgeon (who should be acting as the patient's fiduciary) to the patient herself."

Wall and Brown even used sarcasm. They said that ACOG apparently thought that the signing of an "informed consent" document would be some kind of *"universal disinfectant"* that absolves the surgeon from any responsibility for what might happen to the patient afterward.

The ACOG Practice Bulletins group had "abandoned" its duty "to be an advocate for patients."

Here is what Dr. Margolis had to say about AUGS and this outlandish situation:

1. If AUGS is in the "fray," it is because it intentionally put itself there by its leadership that was rotten to the core being made up of industry whores.
2. If AUGS doesn't want to be in litigation, it shouldn't write Position Papers penned by industry lawyers for use in litigation! (See Nager deposition).
3. This org has never been evidenced based, so don't pretend to be something you're not.
4. You want credibility? Stop taking contributions, grants, honoraria from industry.
5. You want a "new" advisory committee with credibility? Insist that none of its members have any financial ties to industry.
6. Real credibility? Bar any member from serving as an officer of your org from having industry financial ties.
7. It ain't that hard to do. Why can't they see it? Get off the industry tit.

ACOG IN A WHEEL

To understand the high stakes in the "experimental" controversy, you must understand that the American College of Obstetricians and Gynecologists takes itself very seriously. Its website says at the top "Women's Health Matters."

ACOG, like AUGS, is an important part of the medical industry and a strong lobby in Washington. ACOG has traditionally had an influence in board certification standards and processes.

Ob-gyns around the country try each year to earn the status of ACOG "Fellow," doing additional studies and exams with the association. ACOG's annual ceremony inducting new fellows and giving special awards to key physicians does not skip the pomp and circumstance. There are flowing green robes and elaborate ribbons, the traditional Oxford mortarboard cap with tassels.

ACOG holds several important meetings each year, a number of which involve formal-dress dinners, and according to one attendee, "excruciating" cocktail parties where doctors network "intensely" with ACOG leaders who could elevate their place in the elite community.

Both ACOG's and AUGS' huge annual conventions and international conferences are sponsored—underwritten—by drug and device makers. The AUGS conference scheduled for Nashville in 2019 confers Platinum-level status on donors with a $175,000 contribution. (There are also Gold and Silver levels for lesser gifts of $150,000 and $125,000, respectively.)

Here's what $175,000 gets a Platinum sponsor:

- Four 10'x10' booth spaces (20'x20')
- One Industry-Sponsored Educational Session at a Lunch, in which the company can pitch its research and products
- A bag insert to promote the Industry Sponsored Educational Session
- Unlimited exhibit-only registrations and 10 full meeting registrations
- Four invitations to the Joint Presidents' Reception

- Select one: Mobile App/Charging Station/Stacking Blocks (two sets of three)
- Select one: Column Clings/Full-Page Cover Ad in Final Program/Walking Map
- One Registration Bag Insert
- Premium recognition in the Final Program and meeting website
- Premium logo recognition via walk-in slides, signage and booth signage

By comparison, a Gold sponsor at $150,000 only gets two booth spaces, one Industry-Sponsored Educational Session that takes place at an early Breakfast, and three invitations to the Joint Presidents' Reception. They can still get a Registration Bag Insert.

Associations and their patrons take advantage of these conventions to nurture close relationships that produce many companies' KOLs, consultants with lucrative contracts and research grants.

The mesh craze of the 2000s drove up incomes for urogynecologists and then for ob-gyns, and their respective medical societies were among the beneficiaries.

When the word "experimental" popped up in that ACOG bulletin, it jeopardized everything.

A MAJOR VICTORY . . . FOR WHOM?

A trove of internal memos and emails between ACOG members and the largest mesh makers was revealed in 2014 as part of the lawsuits and national litigation against the companies. They show the importance of the "experimental" issue to "stakeholders," and who played key roles in getting the offending word cut.

As soon as ACOG's initial Practice Bulletin with "experimental" came out in February 2007, it set off alarms. On February 5, the chair of the Providence Health system in Oregon sent a note to its OB-GYN department members about the "important ACOG statement on pelvic floor mesh kits." It cited the "potentially serious implications" of the "experimental" nature of POP surgery.

> "I believe the best defense is a great offense. This strong undercurrent fed by the 'anti-mesh' FEW but influential and very outspoken needs to be faced head-on."

In the note, the chair reminded readers of a presentation just a year earlier by one of the founding members of AUGS, Dr. Donald Ostergard. He was concerned with "the lack of long-term data on risks and efficacy" and information on a number of "disappointing outcomes" for patients. Both insurers and malpractice carriers might hold physicians "liable" for injuries in mesh surgeries if the implants were considered "experimental," Ostergard had said.

The chair's note ended ominously: "Even if one does not perform these procedures, (Ostergard's) presentation is instructive to all of us."

That email bounced immediately to the corporate offices of Johnson & Johnson. On February 6, 2007, at 8:07 a.m., Price St. Hilaire, the worldwide marketing director for the Women's Health & Urology division, forwarded that note in an email to Dr. Vincent Lucente, one of the corporation's top vaginal mesh proponents and preceptors.

"Vince, the following email was sent to me from a (company) rep in Seattle . . . Apparently, as a result of some of the discussion at AUGS on industry and empirical data, hospitals are concerned from a medical-legal standpoint."

St. Hilaire asked, "Let me know your thoughts."

Dr. Lucente responded. "I believe the best defense is a great offense. This strong undercurrent fed by the 'anti-mesh' FEW but influential and very outspoken needs to be faced head-on." Lucente urged a written appeal to ACOG for a retraction signed by "every physician in the country" who believes in mesh.

Lucente suggested a female doctor with "no strong industry ties" as the front for the appeal to ACOG. "I am not worried much by the medical-legal aspect as I am by payers who love to use the term 'experimental' as a reason not to pay," he wrote, adding, "BIG problem."

News about the "experimental" label pushed AUGS, ACOG, and mesh makers into "crisis management" mode, as they scrambled to downplay the controversy, while simultaneously fixing it.

Ethicon's medical director for its Women's Health & Urology division, Dr. David Robinson, knew about increasing questions from ob-gyns and urogynecologists about the impact of "experimental" on their practices. On March 20, 2007, Robinson emailed Price St. Hilaire and others at Ethicon about how to handle worried customers—the doctors.

Robinson said company reps would have to explain to physicians that Ethicon/J&J had to keep a low profile. It was critical for the struggle about the ACOG Practice Bulletin to appear focused on science and health, not on revenues.

"Your physician needs to understand that this is not an issue we can be out in the forefront on as it will only appear too self-serving. Our work remains in the background," Robinson wrote.

Ethicon had not sent any formal letter to ACOG requesting a retraction, "nor will there be one sent by Ethicon."

But Robinson wasn't too concerned. He had insider info from the doctors' medical association leaders. "Based on many people's efforts, ACOG is going to be withdrawing the technical bulletin."

Robinson concluded, "It will be re-evaluated and reissued. Hope that helps."

Anne Weber was about to be rolled over by her esteemed colleagues in the urogynecology community. Though the emails continued for a few more months, the battle was already over.

On August 26, 2007, a Sunday, Lucente wrote to his contact at Ethicon, Price St. Hilaire. He was ebullient. "How about ACOG September Bulletin on POP replaces earlier one" from February "and totally 'oks,' vaginal mesh stating . . . 'patient should consent to surgery with an understanding of the postoperative risk and complications and lack of long-term outcomes data' (Duh . . . no kidding).

"Note: No further use of the word experimental!" he said.

"Well, this is one I am taking credit for . . . ," Lucente added. "I led the charge on this and never thought we would get a complete 'replacement' of the earlier bulletin. This is a major victory!"

St. Hilaire responded in the dignified manner of a major health-care corporate executive: "I AM DOING THE HAPPY DANCE!!!! I LOVE YOU MAN!!!!! :)"

> "Well, this is one I am taking credit for . . . ," Lucente added. "I led the charge on this and never thought we would get a complete 'replacement' of the earlier bulletin. This is a major victory!" St. Hilaire responded in the dignified manner of a major health-care corporate executive: "I AM DOING THE HAPPY DANCE!!!! I LOVE YOU MAN!!!!! :)" "With this and the new mesh," he wrote to St. Hilaire, "no tellin how far we can run in 2008 and beyond!"

That evening, Lucente sent another note to St. Hilaire, helpfully suggesting, "Oh, yeah, it may be a good idea to get an email blast out to all sales team" about the excision of the word "experimental."

"With this and the new mesh," he wrote to St. Hilaire, "no tellin how far we can run in 2008 and beyond!"

To be sure, Dr. Lucente was not the only doctor with industry connections throttling ACOG leaders to protect the vaginal mesh revenue stream. But he may have been the highest-paid one. In a deposition for the national mass tort, Lucente confirmed that he had received about $1.7 million from Johnson & Johnson over a period of about 10 years.

Loyalty seems in short supply these days, but over the next dozen years, ACOG and AUGS continued to reliably support vaginal mesh implants no matter what popped up.

A low-key FDA warning about mesh in 2008. A scary FDA warning in 2011. FDA advisory committee meetings. An FDA demand for real clinical trials for prolapse device meshes in 2012. An FDA reclassification of prolapse kits' risk from Class II to Class III.

The message to doctors with that change was: "If you implant this, be really, really careful." The message to mesh makers was: "Find a new line of products." And finally, a recall in 2019 by the FDA of the few prolapse POP kits remaining on the market.

THE LAST LAUGH

Anne Weber continued to oppose AGOG's attack in her Practice Bulletins. In a letter to the *International Urogynecology Journal*, she revealed that doctors in the medical societies were being guided by finances. In fact, the ACOG staff member at the meeting of the Committee on Practice Bulletins—Gynecology described the real reason for concern: "recognition that the current wording would possibly deny payment for some physicians."

"Most of the clinicians who objected to the use of the word 'experimental' understood only too well exactly what meaning was intended," she continued. "Such clinicians were concerned that insurance companies would not cover procedures labeled 'experimental.'"

She went on to slam ACOG, saying doctors should have recognized the fight over the word "experimental" as "a red flag." Clinicians' concerns "were not focused on what was best for the patient, but on what protected their income."

Weber wrote, "That ACOG chose to align itself with these few Fellows at the expense of patients' outcome and safety is of grave concern."

Anne Weber got the last laugh. She became a key witness for plaintiffs in the national mesh litigation, as well as in several state trials.

In a video deposition, she reviewed her voluminous resume carefully and scrupulously detailed the events surrounding ACOG's surrender over the word "experimental." Weber was difficult for defense lawyers to undercut. The MESHdesk report called her a "rock star."

Weber's expertise expanded out from the ACOG controversy. She reviewed data on the problematic Prolift that had been collected and analyzed earlier and shown to doctors around the country. That company-funded research suggested that the failure rate for Prolift surgeries remained fairly low.

When Weber analyzed the numbers, she discovered almost exponential differences in the data that Ethicon/J&J was relying on versus the data as she calculated. Weber testified about the gap, citing in particular one report on Prolift where the failure rate was deemed to be around 2.9 percent. Her calculation came to 27 percent.

Ironically, the doctor whose studies on Prolift were taken apart by Anne Weber was Vincent Lucente.

ROSE KNOWLES'S STORY

When Rose went to Washington in 2007 to testify in Congress about the need for community health centers in rural America, she was managing some 18 clinics in 14 counties across central-western Missouri. She drove about 300 miles per week.

Rose had become the director of Women's Health Services in the West Central Missouri Community Action Agency. She didn't just manage clinic administration, but she was also the free clinic system's advocate in the Missouri General Assembly. "The free women's health clinics were funded under Title X. I filled in as the lobbyist, going from office to office, telling Missouri state senators and members about their constituents and the need for Title X money," she says.

"This is rural Missouri. Many small towns and communities are isolated. Our clinics helped the wives and children of farmers. Most of them had no health insurance." Sometimes Rose went down to the poultry plants to talk with workers about upcoming clinics in their region. "These women had no doctors; they had so little."

The clinics Rose helped were set up in churches, county health departments, schools, county colleges. "Anyone who gave us a place to put our mobile unit and had folding chairs for all the patients who came, we set them up," Rose said. Women got free Pap tests, mammograms, screening for cervical cancer and breast cancer, and a host of other checks and tests.

Congressman Ike Skelton, a longtime representative from Missouri and major player in the nation's capital, brought Rose to Washington to address a hearing in the House of Representatives on the value of, and need for, community health-care centers across the nation's rural areas.

"I was very proud of that work," she says.

Indeed, so was her family, including her youngest son, Mike. "My mom loved her job. She loves helping people. You should have seen all the problems she was handling," says Mike. "My mom was at the top of her game."

On the side, he said, Rose was helping her husband, Jay, fix the budget in their town of Appleton, where Jay was mayor. "She wanted to fix the town's finances; she got Dad to run for mayor so she could straighten things out." The town was in the red when Jay became mayor, but in a few years, Mike proudly shares, it was in the black.

All this action stopped after Rose Knowles got a mesh prolapse kit—Ethicon's Prolift—implanted in 2005. It would upend the next decade of her life.

It's an unusual story, but unfortunately not unique.

To start, Rose did not know she had been implanted with mesh. "I feel ridiculous. Here I was, overseeing health-care clinics for women in the middle of Missouri, and I didn't understand what my own doctor was doing with me."

You see, it started with kidney stones. Rose saw a local doctor for help, ended up with a torn ureter, and still had painful kidney stones. She was told she needed to see a urogynecologist and made an appointment with a leading physician in Kansas City.

"I told him about the kidney stones, what happened with the ureter." Also, she was starting to have a little incontinence when she coughed. "And I was driving across counties where it was 30 miles between restrooms."

After a thorough exam, the Kansas City urogynecologist told Rose that she had serious pelvic organ prolapse—"cystocele, rectocele, everything was starting to sag," he said, according to Rose. "He told me: 'I can help you with that. This situation is going to create more pressure, but we can fix that up.'"

They also talked about her incontinence. "He asked if I leaked when I sneezed; I said yes, but it wasn't my biggest problem. He said I had a total pelvic floor sag and he could fix that," Rose explains.

Rose's mom had pelvic floor sag, too, after bearing 13 children. Rose had only given birth to five, but she thought, now that she was in her 50s, maybe prolapse repair was a good idea. Rose recalled her mom did well after her operation, which involved putting in sutures. "I believed the doctor was going to suture me," said Rose. "I thought that's what I was going to have. How can I explain that I didn't have a clue?"

Around this time, prolapse organ repair, or POP kits, were becoming the Next Big Thing in the mesh industry. By mid-2005, Ethicon was marketing its latest mesh product, the Prolift prolapse kit (without the FDA's clearance).

Rose didn't realize that her doctor in Kansas City was an important key opinion leader, a KOL, for Ethicon/Gynecare— one of their consultants in the pelvic mesh implant business and pelvic floor disorder treatment. He was one of the special pelvic area physicians whom Johnson & Johnson had sent to Sweden in the late 1990s to learn the new vaginal mesh implant procedure for incontinence slings directly from the doctor who had developed it.

Rose felt fine for about a year. During that time her oldest child was diagnosed with breast cancer and passed away. It was no surprise that Rose was devastated and for a while felt lousy, both physically and emotionally.

Then her symptoms started. She had pain in her pelvic area, her bladder was in spasms, and, oddly, there were problems with her right leg. She had trouble walking.

In 2006, she saw several doctors in the Missouri towns where she traveled for work. One told her she had diverticulitis. Another said, "Kidney stones." But those stones had been taken care of, Rose told him. One doctor said she needed a hysterectomy. Another said she had interstitial cystitis.

Finally, Rose returned to Kansas City to see the urogynecologist. But, Rose said, he didn't tell her that her problems might be linked to mesh.

Her conditions worsened. There was searing pain in her pelvic area and in her groin. She couldn't drive as much, and her team picked up the routes for the clinics.

Mike was back home from a tour in the Peace Corps in Central America. "We didn't know what was wrong. She had changed. She was miserable. She couldn't focus. She started missing work and that should have been a fire alarm for us," Mike says.

At another visit to Kansas City, Rose mentions, her doctor seemed frustrated with her situation. He prescribed analgesics. "They made me loopy. They were opiates. I didn't like them." Rose cut back on work because she had too much pain just sitting up, she couldn't walk, and the meds disturbed her concentration.

Rose skipped a family wedding. A special family reunion that she had intended to plan, as she had for years, was dropped. Grandchildren were being born, and she couldn't be at the hospital with the rest of the family because of the pain. And Rose was having trouble urinating.

In 2011, Rose had to quit her job. But staying home didn't stop the pain or the other physical problems. "I found out what people mean when they say they don't want to live," says Rose.

Her son Mike is more blunt: "She became suicidal. When you hear your mom saying she just wants to die, or is ready to commit suicide, what do you do?

"She had been so tough, so strong-willed," he says.

Mike says the family thought it was early-onset dementia. Another doctor suggested she had Sjogren's syndrome, an immune system disorder. Its most common symptoms are dry eyes and a dry mouth. But Sjogren's often accompanies more serious immune system disorders, such as rheumatoid arthritis and lupus. "The doctors were just feeding her pain pills, and that wasn't helping her," he said.

The Kansas City urogynecologist reminded Rose about "the importance of taking all the medications prescribed, and when I was supposed to take them. I told him I did, but he said he seriously doubted that."

The doctor told her to take amitriptyline and gave her shots in her vaginal wall to release the muscles around the area where she felt something sharp coming through. "There were pain pills and special cream I had to use in that area." Rose and her husband had cut back on intimacy because something inside her was scratching him, and it caused her more pain.

In one of the next visits, her urogynecologist said there was inflammation in Rose's bladder causing her urination problems.

"He did not tell me there was mesh likely eroding and moving around," says Rose. Instead, around 2010 or later, he told her there was a new product available that would prompt the bladder to empty itself, and she was a candidate. "I think there was a salesman there in the office that day," says Rose.

The product was the Medtronic InterStim, a device to treat overactive bladders or those with urinary retention. The implant electronically stimulates the sacral nerve, which is thought to normalize neural communication between the bladder and brain.

"When I was in the hospital for that implant, that salesman was there at the hospital; he was giving the doctor instructions," said Rose. "He said that you could adjust the device, turn it up and down," said Rose.

The first time the stimulator went off "I thought I was being shot into the sky," said Rose. And there was terrible pain. She went back to the Kansas City physician and said, "Take it out!"

"He was angry with me," says Rose.

After another unsuccessful appointment a few months later, the urogynecologist handed Rose a referral letter and said, "There's nothing else I can do for you. This is what you're going to have to deal with for the rest of your life. You need a pain management specialist." Then said goodbye.

Rose went to a pain management clinic, and "they started putting fentanyl patches on me. But after a while, I told that doctor, 'I don't want this anymore. I didn't want to live like that, in a big stupor.'

"I went cold turkey on the fentanyl patches," said Rose. "When I told the next doctor about that, he said I could have died stopping the fentanyl that way. I didn't care, I told him.

"I began giving away all my stuff," Rose said.

But one evening she and her husband saw an ad on TV from a law firm about pelvic mesh. "They listed all the symptoms, and my husband said, 'You have every one of them!'" said Rose.

Rose found a doctor, Dionysios Veronikis in St. Louis. He was a well-known removal specialist who had patients flying in from around the world to have their slings and POP kit meshes taken out.

By now, Rose was in a wheelchair because she couldn't

walk. She got in the back of a van, and her husband drove four and a half hours to St. Louis.

Dr. Veronikis examined her and said he knew the mesh had pushed through her vaginal wall and that it had to be removed. "I was in so much pain, my body was screaming. He said, 'That's got to come out very soon, and we will know more when I get in there.'"

The surgery lasted over five hours. "He opened me up hip to hip; the mesh was everywhere," said Rose. "The doctor meticulously pulled out every tiny piece of plastic he could find."

Afterward, Dr. Veronikis showed Rose and her husband pictures from the surgery. "My husband said, 'Now I know what you have been dealing with. I am so angry about what they did to you!'"

Today, Rose is much better.

"I do not take pain meds and I can walk again, though my leg is unstable. I do not have to catheterize myself to pee anymore. I will never be 100 percent since the bladder was badly compromised by the mesh, and I still fight infections. The mesh had worked itself into my urethra, which will have permanent damage," she explains.

In addition, Rose has developed symptoms of a couple of autoimmune diseases that some doctors say are likely linked to the plastic mesh, though that connection has not been proven scientifically.

"How could this happen? I am a fighter, but this almost destroyed me. The mesh migrated and felt like a bowling ball inside of me. It cut nerves in my leg muscles; it was a mess," Rose says.

After the removal surgery Rose checked herself into a mental health treatment center for a couple weeks. "I still could not believe what had happened to me."

"The mesh destroyed my life and all the work I did," Rose shares. By 2015, the free women's health-care clinics across

Rose's 14-county territories were closed. The Title X money had dried up and its proponents had lost the fight for funding. There's still a community action agency, but it does mostly senior care, she said.

"And I'll never get back the income I lost, the cost of all the medical bills.

"I joined one of the lawsuits and I guess people think that if I'm a plaintiff, I must be a real gold digger. Those companies, they thought I was their cash cow. I didn't deserve that."

But at least, Rose says, she's got a second chance.

"My mom lost ten years of her life," says Mike. "She was robbed. Ten years where she would have been making the most money, being most productive financially and socially. And what it did to her relations inside her big family . . . She lost hope.

"The state of Missouri lost an asset too," Mike says. "Those clinics are gone, and she can't bring them back."

But, Mike added, "Mom is definitely trying to make up for lost time."

Rose wants to help other women avoid the injuries and confusion that she endured trying to locate the source of her problems. She says that mesh makers should be held accountable for selling products that could do so much damage: "Women should not be used as meal tickets for the medical industry."

CHAPTER 12

THE HONEY POT

"A society is sometimes judged by the way it treats
its women and children, and I think this was a dark
chapter. These women's lives are altered permanently."

—Dr. Dionysios Veronikis

All surgery has a portion of the unknown to it and is undoubtedly scary, but most of the time we gather our courage and believe that everything will be all right. Actually, that everything will be better than all right since a problem that plagues us will be fixed with minimal healing time. But this is only half of the conversation. We talk to our doctors about the procedure, the recovery time, and what pain meds to pick up from the pharmacy on the way home. However, would we be willing to go under the knife if we fully considered what could go wrong? Do patients understand all the risks that are involved with surgery?

With vaginal mesh, there are two answers that many survivors have echoed over and over again. First, if they chose to have mesh surgery, they were never told of the risks. And second, many were never even told that they were having mesh put into them. These women weren't given a chance to make an informed decision about their bodies because they were never told the full story.

There's also a third group that includes Ceri Baker and many others like her who were given misinformation (a.k.a. lies). During her consultation, her doctor flippantly explained that she could have a transobturator tape (TOT) and that she shouldn't watch the operation on YouTube, "otherwise you'll never do it . . ." There were quite a few women who this hadn't worked for, but he'd done thousands of them and the ones that had problems, he'd managed to sort out. He assured her that it was a simple 45-minute operation that "changes women's lives."

And it did, in fact, change her life: this once-active woman was no longer able to have sex with her husband or ride her bike (her favorite hobby). She's had multiple steroid injections in her vagina and labia, struggles to sit at her desk at work, and needs ibuprofen to get through each day. It wasn't until two years later, when she viewed her medical records, that she saw the letter from her surgeon to her general practitioner stating, "I have discussed the success rate and reoperation risks together with the risk of pelvic organ damage, chronic pain, dyspareunia, and mesh erosion and rejection, but she still wishes to proceed."

This letter shocked Ceri, who adamantly claims, "If any person without a life-threatening condition was offered that selection box of outcomes, would you actually wish to proceed?! . . . [I] absolutely wouldn't have risked all of that for dry knickers!"

NO ANTIDOTE

Like Ceri, most women were never told that this operation can't be reversed. It's not like a Band-Aid that can just be removed or stitches that can be clipped away. Transvaginal mesh is a complicated surgery that is difficult to undo due to the tissue that grows in and around the medical device. While many doctors are able to insert this mesh, few have the training or skill to remove it. Additionally, those who can perform these surgeries may not be able to fully remove the mesh, or they'll need to perform multiple surgeries.

Even with mesh removal surgery, many times the damage caused by the mesh is irreversible. For example, a study conducted by UCLA found that 28 percent of women who had mesh removed said that they had urine leakage at least once a day and half had pain during sex.

And remember how we mentioned that while Boston Scientific and other mesh makers flooded the market with this product, they failed to provide a plan B? Here's why this was a massive issue of negligence on their part.

According to UCLA, "Pelvic organ prolapse (POP) is one of the most common reasons for women to have surgery, with approximately 200,000 inpatient surgical procedures performed for POP in the US each year. A woman's risk of requiring surgery for prolapse is approximately 10 percent. Of those who have surgery, 13 percent will require a repeat operation within five years and as many as 30 percent will undergo another surgery for prolapse or a related condition at some point during their life."

So let's do a bit of math: if 200,000 women in the US have surgery for POP, that means that 13 percent equals 26,000 women who will need a repeat operation in five years and 60,000 who will need an additional procedure. Most of these women were never told that they would be required to have repeat surgeries. Would they have agreed to have mesh for POP if they knew these statistics? Maybe the answer explains why they were kept in the dark.

While thousands of doctors were "certified" to put in vaginal mesh, only a handful are willing and able to remove it due to the delicate nature of this surgery. UCLA explains, "Because transvaginal mesh is considered a permanent implant, surgery to remove the mesh can be difficult and may increase a woman's risk of additional complications or symptoms. Over time, the tissue grows into and around the mesh, so removing the mesh without damaging the surrounding tissue and organs is a delicate process."

"You go in vaginally and take out the mesh there, then you go in through the tummy and chisel out the mesh with some difficulty," states Mark Slack, a consultant gynecologist at Addenbrooke's Hospital in Cambridge, UK. "It's very much not within the skill mix of the vast majority of surgeons."

This is precisely why thousands of women travel to St. Louis, Missouri, to seek the help of Dr. Dionysios Veronikis. Caz Chisholm, 45, from Perth in Western Australia, used a combination of loans, credit cards, and her savings to come up with the $30,000 needed to see the specialist who so many patients affectionately call Dr. V. As Caz told the *St. Louis Post-Dispatch,* "I just decided after all the comments by women about Dr. V, I knew I had to see him," Chisholm said. "No other surgeon would be able to help me."

Dr. V was averaging 30 vaginal mesh removal surgeries a year, but when his patients started sharing their success on social media, his popularity grew. He now estimates that he performs 30 removal surgeries per month. "There's no instructions on what to do when the mesh has eroded in the vagina. I took the approach that it needs to be removed," Dr. V said. "When it becomes infected, it needs to be removed. When you have pain, it needs to be removed."

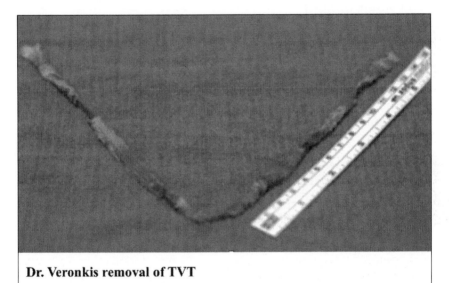

Dr. Veronkis removal of TVT

Unfortunately, complete mesh removal is not always possible. Again, mesh is designed to be a permanent implant and cannot simply be cut out without possibly damaging nerves and tissue. While some doctors claim that they are performing removal surgeries, several are just cutting the loose center piece while leaving the embedded mesh in the body. While this may eliminate a small portion of the problem, the remaining pieces are still sharp and can damage the surrounding areas. They can also cause autoimmune reactions.

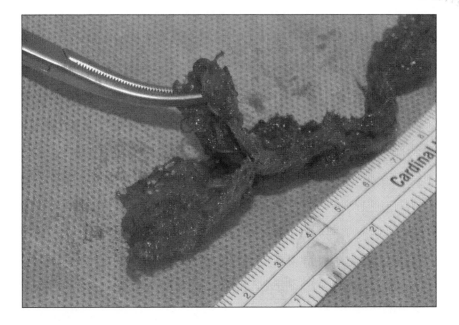

We've also discussed how many different mesh kits were introduced to market and used the FDA's 510(k) application to fast-track products for patient use without testing. Here's another reason why every medical device needs to be tested before going into a person; these small adjustments to create a new product have created another layer of difficulty in removing these types of implants. The University of Colorado Urogynecology department teaches that "if trocars [hook-like surgical tools] were used to place the mesh, as is the case with many commercially available mesh kits, it is often not possible or advisable to remove the arms of the mesh, because they pass through the ischiorectal fossa (a wedge-shaped space in the pelvic area) and/ or obturator muscle. In these cases, we advocate removal of as much of the mesh as possible through a vaginal approach while leaving the mesh arms in place."

Other types of slings used plastic bone anchors that were attached to the pelvic bone to create the correct tension in the mesh sling implant. However, this created additional complications and also made removal difficult if not impossible.

One study conducted by the division of Pelvic Health Center from the University of Washington Medical Center found that "during a

3-year period, 10 patients were referred to us for complications related to transvaginally placed pubovaginal slings using bone anchor fixation . . . The presenting symptoms after surgery included fever, pain, and difficulty ambulating in 1; pain and/or vaginal dyspareunia with discharge in 5; pain or dyspareunia alone in 2; and vaginal discharge alone in 2 patients. Two patients ultimately developed bone lesions on radiologic studies consistent with osteomyelitis. Six patients developed sinus drainage tracts associated with granulation tissue from at least one bone anchor that was unresponsive to outpatient management. One of the patients with pain alone had a permanent suture extending into the bladder neck. Nine patients underwent surgery, of whom five had resolution of their presenting complaint."

Imagine going to the emergency room three times a week for urinary tract infections, undergoing multiple revision surgeries, and paying high prescription prices in hopes that something can take the edge off the pain. Mesh complications have put a huge burden on the health-care system for follow-up treatments and additional care. Billions are being paid out in Medicaid, Medicare, and by private insurance companies. This shouldn't be happening in the US, which has a health-care system that's less evolved and more motivated by money than its counterparts in Canada, Australia, the UK, and Scotland.

MARY'S STORY

"When I was asked, 'What areas of your life did the Mentor OB touch?' I snapped, 'What *didn't* it destroy in my life?'"

Mary is around 40 years old. She was 27 when she had a Mentor ObTape mesh implant for incontinence in 2005. She was happily married, had a young son, a job in a psychiatric unit at a hospital, and was planning on further medical training, perhaps nursing school. She was slender and active in sports, and had a good sex life with her husband.

Today, Mary is divorced. She gave up custody of her son

during their divorce so that her boy could stay in the home he'd grown up in and finish high school with his friends.

The hospital where she worked liked her so much they held her job open for two years after her ObTape implant began to erode. She doesn't work now. She is not in a relationship. She may not be able to have intercourse again. And she limps.

Mary's had 29 surgeries since her implant.

The Mentor ObTape was OK for a while. Mary began having what she thought were female problems, trouble during urination. Then during a night shift at the hospital, her left leg started hurting badly. "By the end of that shift, I was almost dragging my leg," she says.

When she clocked out of her shift, she went down to the hospital's emergency room, got a quick exam. "Inflammation, maybe a pulled muscle," the doctor told her; she was sent home with the anti-inflammatory naproxen.

"The next morning I was in so much pain, I went back to the ER. I don't know how long this went on. I saw my family doctor, a nurse practitioner, went back to our ER two times and then to the ER across town.

"My husband even went in the middle of the night to my parents' house to haul over their recliner because I couldn't sleep in bed; I was moaning so loud," Mary explained.

The doctors did not know what was wrong. They told her it was cellulitis or a pulled groin. "I was athletic, I knew damned well I didn't have a pulled groin." Doctors kept giving her Vicodin and naproxen. "I didn't need pain pills. I needed to find out what had happened to me," Mary says.

Finally, one day when Mary had been sent home again from an ER without an answer or any relief, her sister bundled her into a car and drove some 50 miles away to a major medical hospital in the Midwest. They went into the ER there.

"By that time, my left leg was so swollen that when they measured it, the left thigh was within a couple centimeters of being twice as large as my right thigh," Mary said.

And, she said, "There was a terrible smell—like something was putrefying."

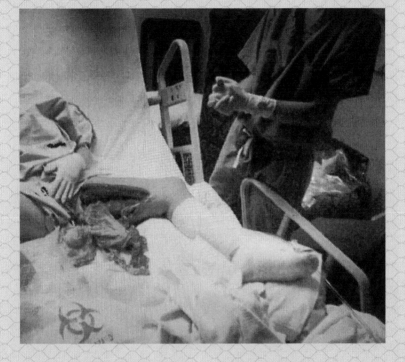

After 45 minutes in the ER, doctors told Mary's sister to contact her family members and get them to come to the hospital. Surgeons were going to need someone's approval to sign an agreement so they could amputate her leg. The problem was an extensive infection in her thigh near her groin. They didn't know the cause, but had to operate quickly.

The doctors saved Mary's leg. However, they had to cut it open from her inner groin to her knee. "You know those Folgers coffee cans? They filled the equivalent of 1½ times the contents of those cans with the flesh and liquid they took from my leg."

The infection was diagnosed as necrotizing fasciitis. Doctors still weren't certain of the cause. But Mary had a flesh-eating bacteria that was very hungry. The infection didn't respond well to initial rounds of antibiotics. At one point, Mary was put in an induced coma.

Then, a doctor familiar with vaginal mesh stepped in. He operated on her pelvic area and found disintegrated mesh. Implanted at the obturator foramen, near the top of the leg, the rotting plastic had migrated and flesh started to fester in her thigh.

"Of course I was surprised. The mesh was supposed to be in my pelvis," Mary said.

The surgery took days. "They said they were going to get out all the mesh, and found many pieces. If they pulled on it, it fell apart into strings, and they had to look for the plastic threads." The mesh was covered in bacteria, she says.

In France, Dr. Michel Cosson heard about this medical case. "That's an example of why I wanted the company to publicize the problems with the ObTape," he said in an interview.

"So that if a woman went to the ER with a fever and infection, especially an infection in her leg that couldn't be explained, doctors would know to ask if she had mesh in her. It would save time. It would save lives."

After so many medical treatments for the wrong condition, Mary started to heal. But it would take several years for her to live a "new normal."

"I'm lucky," Mary says, "I still have pain in my leg, but at least I still have a leg to have pain in. If that doctor hadn't guessed mesh was involved, I might have died.

"I was bitter for quite a while," Mary says. "You feel your physical capabilities dropping off, your mental capacity draining away. It was the only thing in my life.

"I was robbed of my son's childhood," she adds. Her son was five or six when she had the Mentor mesh implant. He was a senior in high school living with his father by the time all Mary's medical and legal issues wrapped up.

"I was at rock bottom. I wanted my son to have stability at that age. And I didn't have any fight left in me. My wounds were healing, but I was still on medicine."

"I had to learn to walk again. Doctors had to cut the muscle out of my leg that you use to pick your foot up off the floor," Mary explained.

One day at a local gas station, Mary says, she saw a young woman, maybe 20 years old, coming out of the station's quick-shop section. "She was drop-dead gorgeous, smiling, and just about skipping. I was so envious. Jealous."

And then Mary saw that the girl was wearing a prosthetic. She was missing a leg.

"It just hit me. I was ashamed. If that girl with one leg could be so happy, moving so easy—with such a smile . . . It was a turning point. I wish I knew who that girl was. What she did was worth a million bucks to me. I'll never forget her smile."

The moment changed Mary's attitude and her relationship with God, she says. And her grown son is now her best friend.

Mary says, "They told me I'd never walk again without a walker or crutches. But I can cross short spaces. I survived this. Don't tell me what I can't do."

FROM BAD TO WORSE

So how far will one of these companies fall to keep their product on the market regardless of the dangers posed to women? Not only will they put volatile mesh into women, which is bad enough, but they're willing to smuggle in cheap Chinese counterfeit materials, too. (And doctors are still willing to use these products and tell their patients that they're "safe.")

Since the early 1990s, Boston Scientific has used Marlex HGX-030-01 Polypropylene Homopolymer resin for its mesh products, and this specific mesh is what was used during the FDA approval process. In 2003, Chevron Phillips purchased the company that was supplying

Boston Scientific's polypropylene, Phillips Sumika, and started asking questions about what the plastic was used for. This was bad timing for Boston Scientific in that they planned to launch a new vaginal mesh product called the Advantage mesh kit and needed several thousand pounds of the material. By 2004, Chevron Phillips issued a warning that it must not be used for "permanent implantation in the human body."

> "I can't, in my wildest imagination, imagine anybody that's knowledgeable in the science of plastics ever deciding that it was appropriate to use polypropylene in the human body. It's well known that its oxidatively unstable."

In an interview with *60 Minutes*, Duane Priddy, a leading plastics engineer and a fellow of the American Chemical Society, explains why polypropylene should never be used in the human body: "I can't, in my wildest imagination, imagine anybody that's knowledgeable in the science of plastics ever deciding that it was appropriate to use polypropylene in the human body. It's well known that its oxidatively unstable." He explained that oxygen breaks up polypropylene, and that although plastic antioxidant additives are used, they dissipate over time. "Once those antioxidants are consumed, they're no longer there to do their job; polypropylene will rapidly disintegrate and fall apart."

The subject of the breakdown of polypropylene mesh is crucial in understanding the long-term damage that this plastic can cause the body. In the magazine *Surgical Technology International*, a group of surgeons published an article in which they explored how polypropylene mesh shrinks and breaks down in the body using a scanning electron microscope. They explain that "immediately after insertion, an acute inflammatory reaction begins. Neutrophils begin to produce oxidants; oxidation of the polypropylene chains produces free radicals, which cause various events, including depolymerization, cross-linking, oxidative degradation, additive leaching, hydrolysis, and stress cracking. These alterations in the chemical structure of polypropylene are responsible for visibly demonstrable fiber changes such as deep surface cracks, flaking, and peeling of the fibers. The processes noted have the potential to cause chronic inflammation, fibrosis, and mesh shrinkage that may lead to chronic pelvic pain . . . The presence of mesh cracking, even at two years out, shows that there are significant structural changes to the mesh."

In 2005, Chevron Phillips refused to be Boston Scientific's supply of Marlex due to the controversy over plastics in the body and stated: "We are simply not interested in this business at any price." Boston Scientific looked into 20 different companies, all who refused.

> In 2005, Chevron Phillips refused to be Boston Scientific's supply of Marlex due to the controversy over plastics in the body and stated: "We are simply not interested in this business at any price." Boston Scientific looked into 20 different companies, all who refused.

And here's some food for thought: in 2007, Boston Scientific contacted Jarden Applied Materials to try to purchase their resin. Boston Scientific sent a list of biocompatibility testing to the company to prove that their surgical mesh was safe for permanent use. This minimal study involved rabbits and was the paperwork that they submitted to the FDA regarding the safety of Marlex as a permanent implant in the human body. While the FDA accepted these reports, Jarden rejected them and refused to fill Boston Scientific's order for implantable surgical mesh. In 2010, Boston Scientific contacted manufacturer Borealis, who also declined, commenting that "they will not knowingly sell their product for use in a medical device."

With the Boston Scientific supply of resin predicted to be exhausted by 2012, they readily made an agreement with a contact in China named Ying "Michael" Zhao and decided to order 30,000 pounds. Now this is where the story gets really interesting. Zhao can't find the certificate of authenticity for the Marlex resin, but he insists that the photo he sent the buyers is Marlex HGX-30-01 and was made in Texas by Phillips Sumika. By September 2011, Todd McCaslin, the director for global sourcing at Boston Scientific, starts to panic because he can't trace the product number back to Phillips Sumika, and Zhao explains that they can't trace the lot number and who the distributor is because the product has changed hands too many times. Boston Scientific proceeds with equivalency testing of the product in November 2011, and the report states that the "results are acceptable even though they do not meet the expected results."

According to plastics engineer Chris DeArmitt, who researched Boston Scientific for one of the women suing the company, "They analyzed 11 different parameters, looking at the two plastics side by side, done, the same tests. Nine of those were different. Two were the same; nine were different. And of those nine that were different, four of those parameters were very different. And somehow, from that, they concluded that it was the same material." Furthermore, one sample proves to have a high rate of titanium.

Boston Scientific's man in China wrote his superiors, "Do we need to ask if this material is supposed to be used in medical implantable?" Boston Scientific's director of materials management replied, "Please don't tell them where we will use it. It could scare them away."

So what does Boston Scientific do at this point? They purchase more of this untraceable, lower-grade material from a shady dealer that will be put into thousands of women's vaginas. The new problem that arises is that the bags are clearly counterfeit. The lot numbers on the bags were fake, the colors didn't match the original packaging from Phillips Sumika, and the city in Texas was misprinted.

Without the proper import records and with bags that were a poor imitation of the original, Boston Scientific knew they had to do something to get past customs to get the 16 tons of goods approved for shipment to the US. This is when Charles Smith, a director in Boston Scientific's Urology and Women's Health division, approved the decision to "overbag" the existing ones, hiding them in plain sight and therefore successfully getting the needed material to create millions of compromised vaginal mesh.

And how would the Chinese product perform in the body? Here's an excerpt from Scott Pelley's *60 Minutes* interview:

> Duane Priddy: I would predict a significant difference in the antioxidant stability, or I should say the oxidation resistance of those products in the human body.

> Scott Pelley: The Chinese product is inferior?

> Duane Priddy: Absolutely. Yes.

> Scott Pelley: Is the Chinese product something that you would imagine being placed inside the human body for 20, 30, 40 years?

> Duane Priddy: Absolutely not.

> Scott Pelley: How long would it likely last?

> Duane Priddy: A few months.

Clearly, plastic doesn't completely dissolve, so what happens to that mesh months after implantation? Like Priddy explains, it oxidizes and breaks down, but before it does that, tissues and veins grow in and around the mesh, making it nearly impossible to remove. When the device weakens, it separates into jagged pieces that can cut nearby tissues, veins, and organs and can even sever nerves, causing leg paralysis. Mesh also shrinks, and with so much tissue encasing it, causes painful pulling, stretching, and other injuries. Additionally, these smaller shards can migrate in the body.

Many complications have been reported for "approved" mesh. This sub-grade Chinese mesh is even more volatile, and while many of us would reject a cheap Chinese knockoff purse or smartphone, how much worse would it be to have an unregulated, permanent medical device that causes crippling pain, inhibits a normal sex life, and creates irreparable damages to internal organs?

> Currently, Boston Scientific is facing a proposed class action lawsuit in West Virginia that accuses it of violating the Racketeer Influenced and Corrupt Organizations Act by selling defective vaginal surgical mesh made of counterfeit supplies from China, reports the *Boston Globe.*

As Americans, we assume that the FDA is there to protect us while closely monitoring what goes into and on our bodies. However, the story of transvaginal mesh paints a clear picture of how the FDA has continually let down the very people it was established to protect. In that study above that took 11 plastic mesh samples and somehow determined that they were close enough to the original resin to be used, the FDA came to the same conclusion, explaining on *60 Minutes* that "we . . . did not find any indication that the change in [plastic] resin led to an increase in adverse events. We have confidence in our . . . findings." They issued a second statement saying that the Chinese mesh "does not raise new safety or effectiveness concerns."

Currently, Boston Scientific is facing a proposed class action lawsuit in West Virginia that accuses it of violating the Racketeer Influenced and Corrupt Organizations Act by selling defective vaginal surgical mesh made of counterfeit supplies from China, reports the *Boston Globe.* The suit seeks unspecified damages for thousands of women who have received the mesh product after September 2012—as many as 55,000 each year.

While the number of patients is mind-boggling, here is something else to consider: at the end of the *60 Minutes* interview, reporter Scott Pelley shared that his team purchased 15 Boston Scientific mesh kits and sent them to a leading plastics lab. All of them matched the Chinese plastic.

CHAPTER 13

SLINGS AND ARROWS

"The pain in my legs and feet was so intense, along with burning pains in my vagina— like being cut with a cheese wire—that I knew something was terribly wrong."

—Kath Sansom, UK

"It's not the surgery; it's the material . . . Now we see what has happened to these millions of women that get mesh . . ."

—Dr. Shlomo Raz, chief of the Urology division of pelvic medicine at UCLA Medical Center

"Biofilm is impossible for antibiotics to kill. The bacteria is covered by a slime, and it's protected from the antibiotics. The biofilm grows, extends, and for that reason patients suffer, five or more years of complications. That includes the systemic complications that we're not told about."

—Dr. Shlomo Raz, chief of the Urology division of pelvic medicine at UCLA Medical Center

In 2018 it was estimated that between three to four million women worldwide had vaginal mesh. As we already know, tens of thousands in America and around the world have experienced terrible damage to their organs from the mesh.

However, countless patients—and even their doctors—are unaware of the link between mesh and autoimmune disease, which causes antibodies to start attacking the body's own tissues. This condition can manifest itself as chronic fatigue, rheumatoid arthritis, lupus, irritable bowel syndrome, and more.

It wasn't until March 2019 that the FDA started to seriously look into the connection between medical devices and autoimmune disorders. "A growing body of evidence suggests that a small number of patients may have biological responses to certain types of materials in implantable or insertable devices. For example, they develop inflammatory reactions and tissue changes causing pain and other symptoms that may interfere with their quality of life," stated FDA commissioner Scott Gottlieb, MD, and Jeff Shuren, MD, director of the Center for Devices and Radiological Health, in an FDA press release.

"Materials used in today's medical devices vary as widely as the devices themselves—whether the material is metal, plastic, silicone, an animal-derived product or some combination of these. Because, in the case of implantable or insertable devices, these materials come into contact with tissue or other parts of the body for sometimes extended periods of time, we do a careful evaluation during our premarket review to determine if there is a potential adverse biological response resulting from contact of the device's component materials with the body and whether the associated risks are unacceptable," the FDA statement added.

A few medical experts have suspected autoimmune reactions to vaginal mesh for years. Shlomo Raz, professor of urology and pelvic reconstruction at the UCLA School of Medicine believes, based on his experience, that 20–30 percent of the complications are what he calls "lupus-type," causing chronic muscle pain, fogginess, allergies—to food, pollen, material—and lethargy. He bases this on the fact that, after removal, the patients are cured of these complications.

"If you remove mesh, and autoimmune-related problems—like the lupus-type symptoms—disappear, the mesh is responsible," Raz said in an interview for this book. He says, "This kind of plastic—you cannot put a lot of it in the human body without provoking response from the body, trying to attack it, trying to reject it." That "rejection" effort is manifested in the autoimmune disease symptoms, he says.

"Some 20 percent of the patients we have seen have what we call "systemic effects," an immune reaction, including hair loss, skin rash, muscle pain, sudden arthritis, similar to lupus-like symptoms," said Raz.

Raz, who has done incontinence implants in the past, says he has tried to limit the amount of plastic mesh in implants. "I never used the precut mesh. I cut my own piece for each patient, and kept it as small as possible."

However, litigation against mesh makers does not allow for mention of any autoimmune symptoms or related problems at all. There are no clinical studies supporting the theory that mesh causes such conditions.

But during interviews with mesh victims in October 2018 in Chicago, the dots connected on autoimmune problems. Women had gathered to protest outside the annual Pelvic Floor Disorders Week conference for the American Urogynecologic Society. For the book, we decided to interview each one separately, so no one would chime in, and they could describe their individual mesh damages.

There were 15 women. Each one of the first five ended their recitation of their mesh damages with "Oh, I forgot to mention—my doctor thinks I've got lupus," or "My doctor wants to test me for lupus," or "I was tested for lupus, and it was positive," or "I was tested for rheumatoid arthritis and lupus, and I have them both."

Lupus is not a common disease. But five out of five of the first mesh victims in our interview list were mentioning lupus. Another six mentioned their doctors' concerns that they exhibited symptoms of lupus before their interviews wrapped up. That's 11 of 17.

Apart from the internal damage from the plastic mesh, several of the women had bumps—big bumps. One woman had them on her abdominal area. Another on her back. They were giant, ugly rashes that were painful and hot.

But the mesh makers still insist there's no evidence that vaginal mesh causes an autoimmune disease.

Clearly, there was a breakdown in the system during the mid-1990s when the FDA determined that plastic mesh was a safe and viable option for vaginal use. But the medical community continues to gloss over the facts and logic regarding mesh-related physical problems, dismissing many complaints by patients they are "treating."

"THE WORST THING THAT CAN HAPPEN TO A WOMAN HAPPENS ALL THE TIME." —REBECCA MEAD, THE NEW YORKER

If mesh were in a man's penis versus a woman's vagina, this disaster would have been blasted into the news as a national catastrophe. Wives would be on TV interviews, sobbing over the loss of consortium with their husbands. The dicks in the medical device companies, greedy doctors, and self-serving lawyers would never have allowed this type of pain and embarrassment to happen to other men.

Here's how Dr. Margolis explains the poor response: "I've seen so many women with mesh who had multiple erosion procedures. The mesh would protrude through their vaginal wall, their doctor would clip it down, and then it would pop up in some other spot. Trying to contain mesh erosion in the vagina is like playing whack-a-mole.

"Let's say they came up with a mesh system for erectile dysfunction. So men who have ED can simply have this mesh wrapped around their penises. This mesh is going to give them better erections, and that's great.

"But then this mesh starts eroding through their penis. And the men have to go through explant after explant after explant, their doctors cutting plastic on the penis again, year after year after year . . .

"How popular would that be?

"I, for one, would find that particularly problematic.

"Just imagine, my doc says: 'Hey, Tom, come back in the office. I've gotta cut some more mesh out of your penis.' I'd say *no* to that idea.

"I guarantee you; I guarantee you: if there was a male equivalent to this shit that caused damage to the penis, this shit would have been off the market about five years before it even came on.

"Maybe it's because you can see a penis and you can't see the vagina. But I promise you, if there was an equivalent mesh implant for penises—that had this erosion, caused pain, male dyspareunia, scarring, dysfunction of the urinary stream—men wouldn't put up with this shit.

"But doctors are doing this shit to women all the time."

IT'S ALL IN YOUR HEAD

The problem is clear: if the FDA has just recently acknowledged this link, then how many women over the past two decades have gone into their doctors' offices, complained of pain, fatigue, brain fog, and more, only to be pushed aside for the next appointment and told that it's "all in your head."

```
doctor: don't confuse
your google search
with my 6 years at
medical school.

patient: don't confuse
the 1-hour lecture you
had on my condition
with my 20 years of
living with it.
```

Many believe that this goes beyond being just a medical issue: it's a gender issue and a modern-day crime against women. For example, let's imagine that Viagra was causing men's penises to decay—like pelvic tissue infected from mesh. This would cause intense pain, which would lead to an inability to work and perform normal daily tasks. It would also eliminate the possibility for sexual intercourse. In much the same way, this is what's happening to women who have had faulty pelvic mesh implanted into their vaginas. Is a woman's vagina worth less than a man's penis? It appears so.

> "It was really clear from the women that they weren't listened to for a long time," explains Chisholm. "It was men making decisions about women's bodies."

In fact, in Australia where TVM prolapse surgery is banned, they are indeed calling pelvic mesh a gender issue. Australian Pelvic Mesh Support Group founder Caz Chisholm fought on behalf of these women and spoke out, claiming that the issue of TVM featured men representing manufacturers defending the devices and male surgeons also defending the devices. However, the victimized women were quieted and grossly neglected for decades to quietly bear their injuries.

"It was really clear from the women that they weren't listened to for a long time," explains Chisholm. "It was men making decisions about women's bodies . . . To the women who have been injured by these devices, it feels like abuse. It feels like a violation. Mesh injury is traumatic and takes the core of a woman's femininity away from her, and the industry is dominated by males."

Hundreds of thousands of women complained to their doctors about the constant stabbing pain, the inability to have sex, and other adverse effects that weren't present before they had TVM, only to be told that these symptoms were "just in their head."

One study has even shown that this discrepancy found in hospitals is standard procedure and explains that women are "more likely to be treated less aggressively in their initial encounters with the health-care system until they 'prove that they are as sick as male patients.'" This bias even has a name in the medical community: "Yentl syndrome."

DEPRESSION AND MESH

As advocates for women suffering from TVM, we've heard countless stories of how these women haven't been taken seriously by their doctors and that they've been made to feel like they're crazy, emotional, hormonal, overly sensitive, and imbalanced. It's not surprising that chronic pain caused by TVM has led to many women struggling with depression.

A study that was published in a January 2019 issue of the journal *JAMA Surgery* was conducted in Canada. It involved 60,000 women in their 20s to 80s who had TVM implanted between 2004 and 2015. From this group, nearly 1,586 of these women underwent surgical revisions. It was found that 11 percent of those who had to have additional surgeries had to be treated for depression and almost 3 percent had engaged in "some form of self-harm behaviour, such as attempted suicide, that led to an emergency department visit or admission to a psychiatric hospital."

"The big challenge with these complications is that in some cases they can be very hard to correct completely," explained lead researcher Dr. Blayne Welk, a urologist at Western University who specializes in incontinence surgery. In an interview in 2019 with the *London Free Press*, he said, "There's an element of decisional regret for a lot of women who have these procedures done. I've seen a lot of patients referred with complications and, a lot of them, they were quite emotional about it and described a long journey trying to find someone to evaluate them and help them with the complications."

Kath Sansom of Sling the Mesh in England knows that feeling of despair. "Women would feel different if they had these injuries from cancer or a car crash. But they are thinking: 'After all, I said OK to the operation.'

"It's a massive head fuck. It messes with women's heads," she said.

"There's a huge journey of acceptance for mesh victims that they've been harmed by something they agreed to. Of course, they didn't know the risks, but still, it's that feeling of guilt—I could have avoided this . . . ," Kath explained.

VAGINAL MESH AND SEXUAL ASSAULT

Can vaginal mesh be considered as a form of sexual abuse and misconduct since thousands—and possibly millions of women worldwide—were put under using anesthesia and then were sexually assaulted by a foreign object that was placed in their vaginas without their informed consent or knowledge? While each state in the US has their own guidelines and definitions, they are fairly similar across the board, but consider that Georgia's definition of aggravated sexual battery is outlined as the following: "intentionally penetrates with a foreign object the sexual organ or anus of another person without their consent." The penalty for this crime is life imprisonment or 25 years' imprisonment followed by probation for life and mandatory sex offender registration.

"Informed consent" is another legal term that we shouldn't gloss over here. According to the American Medical Association, "Patients have the right to receive information and ask questions about recommended treatments so that they can make well-considered decisions about care . . . The process of informed consent occurs when communication between a patient and physician results in the patient's authorization or agreement to undergo a specific medical intervention. In seeking a patient's informed consent (or the consent of the patient's surrogate if the patient lacks decision-making capacity or declines to participate in making decisions), physicians should:

> "(a) Assess the patient's ability to understand relevant medical information and the implications of treatment alternatives and to make an independent, voluntary decision.
> (b) Present relevant information accurately and sensitively, in keeping with the patient's preferences for receiving medical information. The physician should include information about:

1. The diagnosis (when known)
2. The nature and purpose of recommended interventions
3. The burdens, risks, and expected benefits of all options, including forgoing treatment

(c) Document the informed consent conversation and the patient's (or surrogate's) decision in the medical record in some manner. When the patient/surrogate has provided specific written consent, the consent form should be included in the record."

Over the past decade, we've talked to countless women who were never told the risks of vaginal mesh implants; they weren't warned that this was a permanent implant and how full removal is difficult if not impossible, nor were they informed that there were other options available that didn't pose these risks. Of course, we've also heard too many stories about women who never knew they were having mesh at all until they started feeling pain in their vaginas. Danny Vadasz, head of Health Issues Centre in Australia, estimates that there have been 120,000 to 150,000 mesh implants in Australia and approximately 70 percent of the stories his group heard involved a lack of fully informed consent. Many women were never told that a plastic mesh would be implanted into their bodies.

> Of course, we've also heard too many stories about women who never knew they were having mesh at all until they started feeling pain in their vaginas.

So how many doctors have been fined or taken to trial for sexual misconduct or for failing to obtain informed consent concerning mesh patients? *Zero.* Not one doctor has been prosecuted for these crimes.

While these doctors get away with their horrific actions, patients are the ones that have to pay the price every day. Remember when we discussed how there was no plan B? This is where lack of planning, forthought, and compassion becomes the apex of our story as the victims of mesh are now forced to live with the aftereffects of faulty vaginal mesh. Here are some more statements from mesh survivors explaining what life is like for them as they struggle to live each day:

- "The pain in my legs and feet was so intense, along with burning pains in my vagina—like being cut with a cheese wire—that I knew something was terribly wrong."—Kat, UK
- "My children have grown up with a mother who has spent so much of her time in bed, and my intimate relationship with my husband no longer exists."—Victoria, Australia
- "It incapacitated me at a critical time as a mother of three young children and as a wife. There are many things I can no longer do . . . lost opportunities, horrendous medical expenses, bouts of depression, chronic pain and discomfort and continuous bladder prolapse issues. The adverse side effects [I] suffered included bladder dysfunction, nerve pain, mesh erosion, inability to exercise without pain or discomfort, a ruined sex life and an almost failed marriage."—Lucy, Australia

While these stories are heart-wrenching, they are the unfortunate norm of those who are suffering from the intense results of mesh, which makes us wonder, how could this even be legal?

This is what the Centers for Disease Control and Prevention says about sexual violence: "The consequences of sexual violence are physical, like bruising and genital injuries, and psychological, such as depression, anxiety and suicidal thoughts.

"The consequences may also be chronic. Victims may suffer from post-traumatic stress disorder, experience re-occurring gynecological, gastrointestinal, cardiovascular and sexual health problems.

"Sexual violence is also linked to negative health behaviors. For example, victims are more likely to smoke, abuse alcohol, use drugs, and engage in risky sexual activity.

"The trauma resulting from sexual violence can have an impact on a survivor's employment in terms of time off from work, diminished performance, job loss, or being unable to work. These disrupt earning power and have a long-term effect on the economic well-being of survivors and their families. Readjustment after victimization can be challenging: victims may have difficulty in their personal relationships, in returning to work or school, and in regaining a sense of normalcy."

Sound familiar? Genital injuries, psychological problems, inability to work, relational obstacles, lack of normalcy? This is modern-day genital mutilation, only no one is going to jail for these crimes.

"I have seen women with their vaginas essentially mutilated. So scarred and disformed as a result of the chronic inflammation and scarring from the mesh as to be left with a nonfunctional vagina or dysfunctional bladder and urethra," Dr. Tom Margolis explained. "When tissue, the vagina, bladder, or bowel is damaged enough, no surgeon can fix the tissue past a certain point—and I see that with great regularity, even after mesh was implanted years before."

CHAPTER 14

BREAKING BAD

"Puny case settlement values . . .
Successful-in-the-courtroom, surrender-
at-the-settlement-table mass tort."

—Kline & Specter opposition brief to large common benefit payments

"The core of our objection (to large mass legal fees)
is that the cases were settled for way too little and
therefore the lawyers are asking for way too much."

—Shanin Specter, plaintiffs' trial attorney, in Law.com, February 2019

"The women were the losers in this entire process."

—Plaintiffs' trial attorney Adam Slater, 2019

Tort lawyers should have been the heroes of the mesh story.

There are certainly enough villains: greedy mesh makers; avaricious ob-gyns—the "low-hanging fruit"; doctors' associations like ACOG and AUGS; hospitals happily profiting from new streams of revenue in mesh implants; Wall Street; and the device makers' lapdog, the FDA.

But the pelvic mesh mass tort, the largest and most complex in US history, will be remembered as an embarrassing chapter in the history of civil litigation. Many plaintiffs' lawyers joined the list of actors—device makers, doctors, and the FDA—who failed to protect the mesh patients who turned to them for help.

Plaintiffs' lawyers do get a bad rap sometimes. Mass tort lawyers can be arrogant and need serious communication skills training. Then again, they're also the breed that takes on cases on contingency, and they eat what they kill. And without them, the average consumer has no access to the legal system or getting help with their product or drug case.

Part of the growing problem is the "new practice of tort law," not just all tort lawyers themselves. Even some good trial lawyers who look reputable on paper haven't seen a courtroom in years nor have they taken a deposition because of the modern-day tort system, otherwise known as multidistrict litigation or MDL. While this process was created for good reason—to bring swift justice for consumers—it's way too lopsided now with cozy relationships between the lawyers for the plaintiffs and the lawyers for the medical device companies.

In her new book, *Mass Tort Deals: Backroom Bargaining in Multidistrict Litigation*, Elizabeth Chamblee Burch shows how today's plaintiffs' lawyers' interests take precedence over their clients'.

"Your intentions are obvious," wrote a client's attorney to the co-lead counsel for a large mass tort against General Motors several years ago. "You want to control this litigation and maximize the fees earned by your law firm regardless of the harm your actions may cause the MDL plaintiffs."

Burch, the Fuller E. Callaway Chair of Law at the University of Georgia, has tracked the warning signals in several major mass torts. She's found provisions in settlements that benefited the corporations that were being sued and provisions that essentially gave raises to the plaintiffs' lawyers, and she saw the same names appearing as plaintiffs' representations over and over—"the usual suspects."

Currently, Burch is studying how women have been treated in the mesh cases, and her report isn't likely to be positive for the lawyers. In a story in the *New York Times* in July 2019, Burch said publicly what a number of lawyers have been whispering behind closed doors—there was a lack of judicial oversight of the negotiations between MDL teams and the defendant corporations that sell mesh. "You would hope there would be a robust safety net," Burch said. "But there is no built-in review structure to assure fairness." The victims fell "through the cracks."

Protecting "fair" outcomes for victims isn't part of the "new practice of tort law." It has resulted in judges who are not impartial, big payoffs for MDL leadership committee lawyers, and compromised courtroom cases that a lot of them use for meaningless settlements at the settlement table. To make matters worse, the same firms get on the MDL leadership committees, so it's the same forums, with the same political agendas, and they run the game. A lot of these lawyers are located in Houston and have rightly earned the name of the "Houston Mafia."

One problem is that the more the lawyers make, the more they tend to spend on marketing, so the same firms are recycling big money. This gives them the competitive edge on guys who don't have access to the system, even if they moderately try and market. We live in a day and age when people make choices every day resulting from what they see on TV, the Internet, or social media platforms. Consumers look online, visit a website, view back-to-back ads running on TV, and think, "Hmm, they must be good if they can afford advertising."

Good and bad is subjective. Doing well by your client is the pinnacle.

> The women involved pay with mental, physical and financial suffering.

But scalability for a tort that rivaled fen-phen, Zyprexa, and Vioxx blinded some lawyers with dollar signs. They knew they had to be able to go after the universe of hundreds of thousands of cases in a way that they could get enough clients in a settlement to put pressure on the medical device makers. This meant a lot of money for everyone if you looked at the number of cases to be gathered and the net the lawyers billed. Like the rest of the mesh story, the issue became greed.

"America's legal system was set up to help people receive compensation when products or services they bought did not perform as expected. Large settlements that enable firms to address thousands of lawsuits at once work only if the payments go to the right people in the right amounts." The women involved pay with mental, physical and financial suffering . . . In short, it's worth it to everyone to stop this abuse."

BLACK HOLE

In many medical injury cases, particularly when there's heinous product liability, plaintiffs' attorneys have stepped forward to take the place of government regulators (who *should be* protecting patients' safety).

Lawyers sue the manufacturers for product liability or the failure to warn about signature injuries

After a lengthy, torturous, and very expensive process, the lawyers found out what the companies really knew, and when they knew it. Public-minded plaintiff attorneys fight to prevent companies from keeping safety data or incriminating information secret. These lawsuits are often the only way that the public and the government (the Food and Drug Administration) learn that corporations were well aware of the deadly dangers of their products before they even marketed them.

That's how tort lawyers became the last resort for patients, the only way to get reimbursement—justice.

Not this time.

What happened? Scalability. The ultimate mass tort proved irresistible to people who, like device makers and doctors, became greedy.

By 2010, so-called tort reform, a crusade by conservatives and businesses and the US Chamber of Commerce had made headway in their efforts to shut down lawsuits in many states.

In particular, the well-funded campaign cut into malpractice suits. Now there were caps on payouts in lawsuits against doctors and hospitals; some caps were fairly low—$250,000—an amount that might not begin to cover the costs of injuries to a patient. That change forced more tort lawyers into group suits and mass tort areas such as product liability, where the stakes and costs were much higher.

Then in July 2011, the FDA announced a new report on vaginal mesh implants for prolapse. The agency said that over the three previous years its adverse events MAUDE database had accumulated 2,874 new reports of injuries, malfunctions, and even death linked to incontinence slings and prolapse kits.

"The FDA determined that serious adverse events are NOT rare, contrary to what was stated in the 2008 PHN" (the earlier FDA public health announcement on vaginal mesh), the report said, putting the word "NOT" in all capital letters. In addition, the FDA report said, "transvaginally placed mesh in POP repair does NOT conclusively improve clinical outcomes over traditional non-mesh repair."

After the initial thrill about the serious side effects of mesh being deemed "NOT rare" by US regulators, there was a second wave of excitement over the FDA's verdict on the poor relative medical value of POP repair.

In the event of lawsuits, that statement could shoot holes into mesh makers' inevitable claims that POP repair was a critical medical treatment for the "unmet needs" of women with prolapse. If POP repair's value was questionable, then plaintiffs' lawyers could attack the frenzied corporate marketing campaigns to push mesh implants on vulnerable women as just another way to increase profits.

Hundreds of lawyers began looking up "prolapse" and "dyspareunia" and "trocars," or had paralegals do it. The soon-to-be defendants had bragged to investors about the billions in revenue they made in mesh. There were a half-dozen major multinational corporations involved, and dozens of products.

And about two million women in the US had been implanted with slings or POP kits. That meant tens of millions of dollars—maybe hundreds of millions—would be in play.

That is how in 2010 what began with a relatively small "multidistrict litigation" consolidating 36 individual cases across several states involving the Avaulta line of pelvic organ prolapse repair kits—sold by C. R. Bard—led to the addition of more federal MDLs in 2012, 2013, and 2014. Ultimately, seven MDLs were consolidated into one, based in the southern district of West Virginia, whose court is in Charleston. Judge Joseph Goodwin, a longtime jurist with connections to major

West Virginia politicians, was named to oversee the centralized MDL. It grew to include 104,836 filed cases. There were thousands more not filed. The consolidation was a bold move and one that was inevitable. Pelvic mesh cases began to be filed against various pelvic mesh defendants in different federal courts; law firms involved in leadership came together to discuss potential MDL strategies.

One of the obvious issues was the presence of numerous cases where a single plaintiff was implanted with multiple products, involving similar defects and several serious side effects. Mass consolidation of all the pelvic mesh cases and centralization of strategy and judicial rulings was the only way forward. The largest silos of cases were those involving Boston Scientific, American Medical Systems, and Ethicon (a Johnson & Johnson subsidiary), according to court records.

THE USUAL SUSPECTS

When a mass tort—or multidistrict litigation—starts to come together, law firms congeal almost automatically into a legal hierarchy. At the bottom, small firms with minimal or no tort experience help larger firms search for clients and, in turn, receive a finder's fee from the larger legal firms.

"My boss was told there might be some action with this product called vaginal mesh. I was told to start sifting through files of current

> I was told to start sifting through files of current and former clients—car accidents, bankruptcies, clients with middle-aged women—to find possible plaintiffs for this new issue," said a lawyer who was a junior associate at the time in a Midwest firm.

and former clients—car accidents, bankruptcies, clients with middle-aged women—to find possible plaintiffs for this new issue," said a lawyer who was a junior associate at the time in a Midwest firm.

The midsized firms started to skim through information and began to establish potential lists to send along to the largest tort firms, the mass tort "insiders," like those involved in the fen-phen diet-drug saga, Vioxx, hip implants, or asbestos lawsuits.

Savvy lawyers reached out to local doctors to inquire whether they knew any physicians whose female patients had pelvic mesh implants. Some of them even reached out to sales reps for device makers who

> The more claimants a firm had, the more likely the firm was to get a place somewhere on one of the influential committees that would be established to deal with the multidistrict litigation.

sold vaginal mesh to hospitals or medical clinics. "Word gets around, and my job was to start identifying possible clients, women who could have claims," one lawyer said.

Many of the largest firms began a new line of TV and web advertising and created call centers to review potential mesh clients.

But only a handful of firms really intended to get into court. The plan as it unfolded was to amass long lists of clients. The more claimants a firm had, the more likely the firm was to get a place somewhere on one of the influential committees that would be established to deal with the multidistrict litigation. Seats on those committees would become valuable.

This was where numbers counted. Where chips were called in. One participating lawyer likened the operation to the trading that goes on at the NFL Draft.

Each "mini-MDL" would need its own leadership structure reporting to the main MDL. And there were so many different products—TVT slings, single-incision slings, POP kits with different tools and different sizes of mesh. They all needed participating firms that could specialize in a defendant company, plastic materials, or a product.

And, of course, at the top would be the committees of elite tort lawyers set up to manage each MDL. The fee committee would be a prime spot for the "regulars"—the early settlers called Pilgrims, the

> Firms boasted of having 20,000 plaintiffs. But they couldn't actually interview all the patients in detail or learn the extent of their injuries.

Houston–Dallas axis of attorneys known affectionately as the Houston Mafia, powerhouses from New York and Los Angeles. Many smaller law firms cozied up to the veterans, who were obviously going to big players in the mass tort structure and committees.

So many spots to fill, so much money to make.

Lawyers quickly amassed too many clients. They warehoused them. Firms boasted of having 20,000 plaintiffs. But they couldn't actually interview all the patients in detail or learn the extent of their injuries. They could only hope to end up included in one of the mass settlements where plaintiffs' lawyers would ultimately control the grid that determined payments to clients from group payouts.

Eventually, working with judges, there would be a handful of bell-wether cases chosen to go to trial—though that didn't even happen for all the companies. And those bellwether outcomes would affect what each defendant was likely to pay to the combined plaintiffs of the MDLs.

But what about the women?

TIME BOMB

Initially, law firms were committed to getting justice for injured women. But many lost that focus. Mistakes were made. Bad choices followed.

After signing up too many clients, the biggest mistake by the MDL lawyers is that they allowed the defendants—like Johnson & Johnson, Boston Scientific, and American Medical Systems—to set the agenda. It's usually in corporate defendants' interest to drag out mass tort litigation. But with pelvic mesh, it was sometimes in the corporations' interest to settle quickly and move on.

After all, the numbers of potential mesh victims are staggering. If 10 percent of the US mesh surgeries resulted in damages requiring some kind of surgical repair, 10 percent of two million means roughly 200,000 women were potential victims, minimally. We all know it is staggeringly higher.

> The major problems with vaginal mesh, migration and erosion, do not always present themselves within weeks or months of the implantation. Doctors say they are seeing patients whose implant was eight or nine years ago, coming in with terrible pain, uncontrollable incontinence, bleeding. The women were fine during the previous period, examples of patient success stories touted by companies and ob-gyn groups.

From the start, Judge Goodwin made it clear that his focus was speed. And from the way these mass cases were being collected and handled, speed trumped the quest for reasonable compensation for severely injured women, for justice, for accountability.

Over the last decade, the number one mandate in civil litigation is to settle mass torts quickly in order to avoid clogging or burdening the system and to provide swift justice.

The poor, overburdened system. Let's have a moment of silence for the system.

Now let's get back to the victims.

The major problems with vaginal mesh, migration and erosion, do not always present themselves within weeks or months of the implantation. Doctors say they are seeing patients whose implant was eight or nine years ago, coming in with terrible pain, uncontrollable incontinence, bleeding. The women were fine during the previous period, examples of patient success stories touted by companies and ob-gyn groups.

Unlike a number of the devices and drugs that were the focus of national lawsuits and withdrawals from the markets, vaginal mesh has time on its side. With diet drugs like fen-phen or Vioxx, or flawed heart stents, most of the damage appears within months or a couple of years. If the patient doesn't have symptoms of heart valve damage or pulmonary hypertension in the first year or so of taking Redux, their chances are better than average that they will not suffer those damages. If you stop taking Vioxx and other pain medicines in that drug family, your risk of having a heart attack linked to Vioxx drops precipitously. Whatever the outcome, the patient and her doctor know the extent of the injury and the future risks it poses; there are few surprises in store.

Mesh, however, is like a ticking time bomb. According to Dr. Tom Margolis, "The damage can show up years later, and often does."

The delay in the appearance of catastrophic injuries needing major surgery is the critical issue that should have gotten much more attention, and more medical provisions in the MDL settlements. The plaintiffs' attorneys were shortsighted. It was all business as usual.

Tort lawyers should have stressed the delay of months, sometimes years, caused by the failure of doctors to tell patients that their mesh implant was the reason for their pain, bleeding, urinating and sudden or uncontrollable defecation. It's clear from trials and medical records that many doctors did suspect or know that the mesh implant erosion was the source of their patients' injuries. Those physicians should have sent their patients quickly to urologists, not to psychologists, physical therapists, or pain management specialists.

> Big law firms managing the MDLs were busy trying to meet judicial deadlines—and the quicker the settlements, the sooner the money would be available. This was especially important for law firms that had taken out huge loans to advertise; they could not afford to wait around for years for the payouts.

Big law firms managing the MDLs were busy trying to meet judicial deadlines—and the quicker the settlements, the sooner the money would be available.

This was especially important for law firms that had taken out huge loans to advertise; they could not afford to wait around for years for the payouts.

"The synergy between the bottom-line interests of the plaintiffs' lawyers, the bottom-line interests of the defendants, and the interests of the court in getting this finished—it all came together to drive settlements of thousands of cases at a time," says Adam Slater, who worked with the MDL and shared key depositions and discoveries from the New Jersey litigation. He has tried six mesh cases in court, winning tens of millions of dollars.

"A woman whose case had already gone to trial came to me," said Slater.

The woman had not had surgery yet at the time; she was awarded about $50,000 by the jury.

Within a few months, the woman underwent mesh revision surgery. "She asked if I could take her case, get it back to court. But there was no way for me to help her." If she could have waited, she could have gotten a much larger figure that would have paid for her injuries, Slater said. "Her case ultimately was worth much more."

But too many lawyers weren't paying attention to their clients' needs.

"The vast majority of these women were preyed upon by law firms that are marketing and collection firms, and not actual litigation and trial firms," Slater said. "Their business model is bad for seriously injured victims.

"These firms that created a system that had call centers," he said, often people without knowledge of the case manage the paperwork. "The lawyers never meet most of their clients, never talk with them; patients can never get a lawyer on the phone," Slater added.

SYSTEMIC BREAKDOWN

The mesh disaster has highlighted flaws in America's approach to large litigation.

"This mass tort system, which is a sick, anti-client system the way these plaintiff firms run it, where they warehouse these thousands of cases. That was one of the reasons these women were harmed," said Slater. "The entire system conspired against them."

Acceptable complications or injuries must have a causal link to the product like mesh, based on peer-reviewed studies in medical and scientific journals and experts retained for the litigation. The patient's medical records must show she used the product.

And there must be testimony from medical providers that the patient's injuries are similar to those recognized as side effects in medical studies.

There was nothing in the combined cases about side effects involving autoimmune diseases like lupus, which so many women were diagnosed with in the early years after their mesh implants.

Women who had multiple surgeries—and there are thousands of them—were also getting shorted. For example, a number of women had two to four major surgeries to remove mesh from them (some even had 10 or 15). But injuries to organs such as their bladders, urethra, uterus, and obturator nerves required further operations. The additional surgeries did not involve actually "removing" more mesh, but sewing up, shoring up, or removing damaged organs.

"These women with seven or 10 surgeries are being told it doesn't matter that they need their vaginas or urethras rebuilt or replaced. All those other surgeries don't matter," said one of the mesh lawyers. "It's ridiculous."

Some women's damages involved serious and life-threatening infections that spread outside their pelvic area, outside the "migration" of the mesh itself. Surgeries were needed to remove the dead, necrotic flesh and stop the infection. They were forced to battle repeatedly for settlements that covered their extensive injuries because they weren't undergoing "revision," meaning mesh "removal."

Lawyers fought to limit payouts to patients who were hospitalized, not those whose repair procedures were done on an outpatient basis.

Women whose damages were limited to hardened mesh repeatedly protruding through their vaginal wall and injuring their partners during intercourse might not qualify for anything, especially if the repair did not involve a hospital visit. If a doctor "trimmed" the mesh in his office, it was unlikely to pass the "mesh removal" test. Even if the woman had to return several times to her doctor as the mesh continued to migrate.

STATUTES OF LIMITATIONS, OR SOL'S

Over the last 15 years, the well-funded campaigns of the Chamber of Commerce and the American Legislative Exchange Council have decimated tort suits at the state level. One of the targets in tort reform has been to limit statutes of limitation.

But many women with mesh implants did not know the source of their pain or illness because the medical community failed them at many levels. They were misinformed or misled by their physicians and didn't know that they had mesh; the FDA failed to acknowledge a link between autoimmune illnesses and medical implants at this time, and no one thought to create a registry to document patients with vaginal mesh implants. Other devices on the market such as pace-makers, stents, joint replacements, and more are tracked in hospital or health-care databases to monitor "patient safety, quality, outcomes, and cost-effectiveness," according to Kaiser Permanente. However, there was no way for many women to know what type of implant was put inside of them until it was taken out. This means that these women were not told that their pain or bleeding was due to the mesh implant, so they lost months, even a couple of years, bouncing from doctor to doctor to find out what was wrong and to get relief.

That wasn't as much of a concern in states where the statute of lim-itations does not start running until a patient discovers she has been injured by the product at issue, in this case, mesh.

Judge Goodwin did attempt to find paths with some flexibility for victims in time-limited venues, several trial lawyers said. In 2018, during protracted negotiations over thousands of cases awaiting Johnson & Johnson's settlement offer, Judge Goodwin dismissed some 22,000 suits against Ethicon. They involved women who had not yet had revision surgery, the main standard for a pelvic mesh claim to be considered for inclusion in the MDL.

That decision was probably positive. Judge Goodwin dismissed those cases "without prejudice," meaning that they could be refiled later by women whose symptoms worsened and needed an operation. Goodwin basically extended their statute of limitations by giving those patients another five years in which to demonstrate sufficient damage (i.e., requiring "revision" surgery).

MISSING RECORDS

In a nation whose insurance companies, hospitals, and health-care industry are obsessed with collecting detailed data, it was surprisingly difficult for some women to obtain copies of their medical records showing what kind of mesh implants—what brand—were in them.

Doctors' offices don't have to keep medical records forever. But that doesn't explain how a woman whose implant surgery was only five years old could not get her hands on records showing which company or companies' products had been used.

Hospitals were the major buyers of mesh implants, according to former sales reps, and should have known what specific products they were buying. You would think that records of hospital purchases wouldn't just disappear. And knowing the aggressive efforts by major medical device makers' sales reps to establish close relations with their buyers, it seems someone in a hospital purchasing system would have known which brands of mesh products had been frequently implanted.

The mesh makers would certainly know, because the corporations counted every sling and every POP kit they sold, and tracked where they sold them. But getting that information would involve a lot more cooperation by the defendants.

THE AMS DEBACLE

In April 2011, American Medical Systems, which had seen amazing growth and profits with its pelvic meshes like Apogee and Perigee, was bought by Endo Pharmaceuticals for some $2.7 billion. The announcements at the time cited AMS' female incontinence products as a factor in the acquisition. Three months later the FDA issued its warning that serious side effects from pelvic mesh were "NOT rare." Within two years, AMS was foundering under the mesh litigation.

There hadn't even been a trial yet involving an AMS vaginal mesh implant when AMS proposed settling tens of thousands of cases. It was a good move for the company, but the ramifications for victims— not only AMS' victims—was a disaster.

In polite terms, the AMS litigation was "too immature" to be settled, according to Philadelphia attorney Shanin Specter of Kline & Specter. But AMS dangled the threat of bankruptcy in front of the MDL, he said.

That caused a little panic among the lead lawyers for the MDL. In 2013, Endo, which had bought AMS, settled an undisclosed number of mesh cases for $54.5 million, according to Reuters. The following April, it settled another 21,700. And in September 2014, Endo announced it would settle another 20,000, ending nearly all the US cases against AMS. The company would increase the amount of money set aside for mesh claims from $1.2 billion to nearly $1.6 billion, Reuters reported.

Nonetheless, women came out short. The bankruptcy threat by AMS lawyers scared the MDL into accepting too little funding in the settlements on behalf of the clients.

> Nonetheless, women came out short. The bankruptcy threat by AMS lawyers scared the MDL into accepting too little funding in the settlements on behalf of the clients. Today, the companies that own AMS, and its top executives, are doing just fine.

AMS told the MDL leaders, "Look, this is all we'll be able to pay you." So other firms went to AMS and said, "We'll take that too, rather than take nothing," Slater explained. The lawyers had inventories of so many cases that were not going to be compensable and were saying, "What are we going to do, AMS' stock is going down, we're worried, we can't wait," Slater added.

Today, the companies that own AMS, and its top executives, are doing just fine.

THE TRICKLE-DOWN EFFECT

"The whole judicial system failed these women, not just their lawyers," said Slater.

AMS' low-value settlements quickly began to seep into other MDL litigation. The basic problem, according to several plaintiffs' attorneys, was that the focus in the MDL was to *settle* the cases; that was Judge Goodwin's mandate. That's all fine if you're going to try to get "fair values" for your clients.

But when a large group of lawyers settled with AMS early on, and settled for values of $40,000 a case, taking even $25,000, that then became the "market" for mesh cases in the MDL.

It didn't matter that AMS' claim that it was going out of business had caused the plaintiffs' lawyers to take the "puny" settlements, as they were later called by one angry attorney who was part of the MDL. Boston Scientific, Bard, and J&J began pushing hard for "low-ball" settlements, too.

The pressure from the court on the MDL plaintiffs' attorneys intensified. Lawyers were urged to move faster to end the larger litigations as for Boston Scientific.

The firms that were warehousing cases got a boondoggle. Suppose a firm's fees from a low-settlement client come in at a mere $10,000. If that firm has 500 similar cases, then it makes $5 million.

What about firms that had inventories of 1,000 or 5,000 or 10,000 cases? Do the math—MDL lawyers certainly did.

Now the tale takes a downturn—yes, now. Surely in a group of 500 cases there were women with catastrophic damages whose settlements were worth far more than $40,000 to $45,000? Why push those victims to take such small amounts?

Because many firms that boasted high inventories of cases did not actually interview their clients. Some women signed up with a firm and years later still had not talked with "their lawyer" or any lawyer at the firm. And the firms had too many clients to get involved in demanding all the records from hospitals and doctors, so a number of women on claimant lists had no proof they had a specific company's implants. State time statutes were ticking away, and a number of women who were still waiting to have a conversation with "their attorney" were going to be out of luck.

Why? Some firms with large client inventories did not anticipate the speed with which Judge Goodwin was moving the various MDLs.

In 2014, Judge Goodwin set up "waves" for claimants' cases to start moving forward. He worked chronologically, so the oldest implant cases moved first. Goodwin informed MDL leaders that he expected cases would be filed in the appropriate state courts, and lawyers would be prepared to begin discovery, take depositions, enter motions, and generally be waiting for the started pistol to fire. Their cases would probably not get to a trial, but they had to get ready within, say, two months.

Suddenly, "warehouse" lawyers began calling around, asking other attorneys what to do.

How would they tell their client: "I'm suggesting you take the settlement, because I can't handle all these cases, because I took too many cases." That might be awkward.

> Many women wanted to reject low-settlement offers, but were coerced to concede. Their lawyers sent them formal letters giving a dozen reasons to take the settlement. And then they added, "If you don't take this settlement, we're not going to represent you anymore. You can find a new lawyer."

And what would the lawyer tell Judge Goodwin? "I can't meet your deadline to work up my cases because I have too many, or I haven't even started working on the file?" That's saying you can't fulfill your obligations to your client.

"It's a serious, serious problem with the system that they were allowed to just collect thousands of cases," said Slater.

Many women wanted to reject low-settlement offers, but were coerced to concede. Their lawyers sent them formal letters giving a dozen reasons to take the settlement. And then they added, "If you don't take this settlement, we're not going to represent you anymore. You can find a new lawyer." But so many years later, they had no options because most law firms would no longer take older mesh cases.

A number of women interviewed for this book received such letters. "You don't know what to do," said one woman with catastrophic, permanent injuries. "And none of these lawyers want to sue another for malpractice on my behalf," she added.

Shanin Specter remembers the panic that began when Judge Goodwin decided to move the mesh cases forward, one tranche at a time. "I had conversations with a number of the lawyers in the mesh MDL, including some friends who have large inventories," he said.

"One lawyer was candid enough with me to admit he had taken on too many cases and boxed himself in. When the MDL 'waves' started pushing cases forward for resolution, he couldn't handle discovery for all his cases.

"He reached out to me," Specter continued. "He really wanted to litigate them, and try many of them. But he became overwhelmed. Therefore, he had to accept an inadequate settlement."

Specter said he doesn't have a problem with lawyers taking lots of cases, even in four figures. But he thinks that 8,000 to 10,000 are too many to handle. "Just look at all the money spent on advertising by lawyers," he said. "When a poor settlement is put on the table, the one fact that a plaintiff's lawyer should *not* be considering is 'How many clients do I have?'"

Mr. Specter's firm has a winning record with mesh trials in Philadelphia; in January 2019, client Suzanne Emmet, who was implanted with Johnson & Johnson's Prolift, won $41 million. Specter has more scheduled for 2019 and 2020. "A lot of cases were tried in court, and they've been overwhelmingly favorable to the clients," Specter said. "Of 32 cases, 24 verdicts have gone to the plaintiff." The average jury verdict over the last two years is close to $20 million, even discounting a judgment to knock down the amount awarded in one of them.

In fact, the first bellwether case for the MDL was a win for the plaintiffs. After an excruciatingly long and hard-fought discovery process, Judge Goodwin set a trial with four plaintiffs, *Amal Eghnayem et al. v. Boston Scientific*. Each of the women claimed they had suffered severe damage from the company's popular Pinnacle kit for prolapse.

It was cold and rainy in November 2014, back in West Virginia, where the main MDL was based. Judge Goodwin transferred the case to Miami and presided over it himself. The trial took eight days, but the jury needed only one to return a verdict: the four women together were awarded a total of $26.7 million.

If the mesh cases weren't so successful in court, or juries awarded too small amounts to plaintiffs, it would be one thing, said Shanin Specter. But the trials' results show that the amount in settlements could be more significant for the plaintiffs, he added.

Only about 20–30 percent of the total cases could be tried because of statutes of limitation and causation issues. "But even with that, you can't settle these cases for $40,000 each and think you're doing a good job for your client," Specter said.

Specter raised the example of the Vioxx litigation, an MDL created in the wake of reported heart attacks and other cardiac events linked to the prescription painkiller made by Merck. It was withdrawn from the market in 2004. Only 12 of 17 trials got verdicts for the plaintiffs, and five were overturned, he said. However, "Vioxx was settled with an average of $100,000 per client." There were about 50,000 claims, and Merck put up $4.85 billion. "The settlement of $100,000 was very reasonable in that light," Specter added. And the legal fees were capped at 32 percent, he said.

Like several other lawyers interviewed, Specter says the AMS settlement was premature. "We settled with AMS because of their financial jeopardy, but we didn't really get fair values," he stated. He has a warning for future settlement offers: "So, no more breaks because of financial problems. Look, AMS has rebounded. NO MORE BREAKS."

WAR STORM

Around Thanksgiving 2018, Kline & Specter dropped a bombshell in the MDL litigation. As most of the companies have preferred settlements, the time had come for the MDL leadership to divvy up the monies that had gone into the common benefit fee fund. Kline & Specter filed a brief objecting to the proposed common benefit haul of at least $336 million.

The brief castigated the MDL for failing to arrive at a global settlement for the mesh victims. "Most settlements were wholly inadequate, considering the seriousness and permanence of their injuries," the brief said, citing the average of approximately $40,000.

"Puny" was what the brief called the MDL's settlements, an adjective that did not sit well with the MDL's fee committee.

The brief also noted that courtroom trials demonstrated how much more money the MDL should have demanded in negotiations from the defendant corporations, suggesting MDL attorneys caved. It described the MDL litigation as a "successful-in-the-courtroom, surrender-at-the-settlement-table mass tort."

When asked later about the slash-and-burn brief by Law.com, Mr. Specter gave a simple explanation. "The core of our objection (to the fees) is that the cases were settled for way too little, and therefore the lawyers are asking for way too much."

Judge Goodwin didn't agree with Kline & Specter, and in February, the Law.com headline read: "Judge Grants Potential $550M in Pelvic Mesh Fees, Allocation Fight Looms." The common benefit fee fund that had been around $336 million just a few months earlier was now speeding past a half billion dollars.

That spring, Adam Slater's firm Mazie Slater Katz & Freeman complained about the allocation of the MDL leaderships, noting that he and his group had produced depositions from key witnesses. But Judge Goodwin rejected their complaint, too.

Still, both Kline & Specter and Mazie Slater Katz & Freeman received payment from their common benefit fee funds for their roles in the MDL.

"The *women*, particularly the most severely injured women who were represented by law firms that never intended to seriously litigate their cases, were the losers in this entire process," said Slater.

CHAPTER 15

MESHED UP

"Women that have had those implants, who have
those outcomes . . . have been failed in a monumental way by the system and by certain people in the medical profession who they trusted. I
hope that we never have to have another inquiry
where we see such suffering from the witnesses."

—Senator Rachel Siewert to the Australian Senate

While American women were dealing in relative silence with the
"complications" from vaginal mesh implants, mesh patients in the
Commonwealth were making noise.

There were loud arguments in London in Parliament over the injuries to British women from mesh. The National Health Service worried
the cost of repairing or removing eroding mesh from women could
cripple its finances. Several major newspapers and the *British Medical
Journal* conducted investigations of the mesh craze and what the companies really knew about their products. A baroness met with mesh
victims all over England to hear about their injuries.

The Scottish Parliament asked an American tort lawyer to address
them about mesh dangers and what he'd found in manufacturers' confidential corporate records.

Ireland announced plans to limit mesh surgeries.

Australia banned POP kits and the single-incision mini-slings in 2017. Its Senate conducted an investigation on mesh and published it in 2018. Australia's health minister issued a public apology to the women of the country for what had been allowed to happen to them.

And in April 2019, Australia's third-most populous state, Queensland, opened a special clinic for the integrated, holistic treatment of mesh injuries. It's funded by the government. And it was co-designed by a number of the mesh victims whose assertive advocacy made mesh an issue that Australian politicians could not ignore.

How did this happen?

The high profile of pelvic mesh problems in the UK and Australia comes down to the women who refused to sit down and shut up.

Using Facebook and other social media networks, women organized grassroots activism.

They ran savvy public interest campaigns from their living rooms to air their grievances. Their homegrown movement actually upended the well-financed pushback from some of the biggest international mesh maker corporations and their lobbyists. These women's efforts had national impact on the regulation of vaginal mesh implants.

SLING THE MESH

In Britain, Kath Sansom drove the movement forward through her website Sling the Mesh.

It was 2015 when Kath Sansom had a TVT incontinence sling implanted. She was 47, with two children—the second had been a difficult birth. She started leaking while doing high-impact exercises at the gym. "I'm a fitness fanatic," she said in an interview. "I should have just had physiotherapy to control the incontinence."

Instead, there was a sling procedure followed by "unbelievable pain." She couldn't find out why she was in such distress, or if anyone else had similar problems. Kath found another woman online who had mesh pain, and began her march.

She connected with more mesh victims, ones who got the same kind of brush-offs that women in the US were getting when they complained about the implants. "It's in your head." "It's menopause." "It will go away soon."

One of the side effects, LUTS—lower urinary tract symptoms—didn't register with doctors. "They say: LUTS is nuts," Kath said. And so doctors were sending women with chronic urinary tract infections home without any antibiotics. "And the women had to return to their physicians with the same symptoms "all the time," added Kath.

"Women were going back and forth to doctors for years after their implant, thinking their problems and pain were just cystitis, because that's all their doctors told them."

She said, "People don't understand how serious these mesh injuries are." But some women did.

Only 10 weeks after setting up the Sling the Mesh site, "we had more than 7,500 members globally. We even have logos and banners now," Kath said.

Kath says the response to her site showed that there were many women with more serious complications than doctors or health officials or the companies were telling the public.

"The first thing we needed to do was engage the media" in coverage of the mesh issue, Kath explained. That's when she saw the influence of male editors in male-dominated newsrooms. "They didn't want to talk about any of this. They were almost giggling, laughing at it when we talked with them."

Kath told the men it wasn't funny. "It's a *global corruption* story."

"It took about a year to break them down," she says. The *Guardian* and the *Daily Mail* began running stories about individual women whose lives had been upended by mesh, and that prompted more coverage. "Now we can talk about vaginas, prolapse, mesh, problems during sex . . . ," Kath says.

"I just kept telling these women's stories, getting their stories into magazines and daily newspapers," said Kath. Women have suffered in silence too many years, she said.

As with the thalidomide scandal in the 1960s, "I decided that I'm just going to keep telling the story over and over again until they 'get' it. Like the editor of the *Times*, they had to hear it again and again."

The campaign got boosts from the *Victoria Derbyshire* TV show in Britain, SKY UK, and the *Daily Mail*, among others.

Labour politician Owen Smith, a former journalist, got it. "He encouraged women on my site to channel their action into contacts with their [Parliament] members," said Kath. That effort accelerated. "We were getting women to email or mail their MPs, the National Health Service, medical groups," demanding a public accounting of the damages caused by the pelvic implants. It created political pressure.

> And some politicians started questioning the easy medical device approval system that imposed tougher standards for toasters than for products placed in British women's vaginas.

Once the patient stories were showing up regularly in national and local media outlets, reporters turned their attention to the issues in the National Health Service and with the mesh makers. Most importantly, the media, including medical writers, began writing about the gap—a chasm, really—between the sunny picture of mesh patients painted by the companies (and UK physician groups) and the terrible pictures of injured women.

The National Health Service began reporting about the real rate of surgical "complications," at one point saying that serious side effects were showing up in as many as 15 percent of the women who had mesh implants. The NHS had good data because it was paying for the repairs, including removal surgeries.

Meanwhile, the Royal College of Surgeons called for a "compulsory" national registry of mesh implants in patients. And some politicians started questioning the easy medical device approval system that imposed tougher standards for toasters than for products placed in British women's vaginas.

And in the middle of all this was the Sling the Mesh network, chronicling each news story and each meeting, nudging along politicians, using its website and Facebook page.

On April 19, 2018, the House of Commons held a debate on the problems with vaginal mesh implants. The pre-debate package assembled by the Backbench Business Committee laid out the issue and supporting documents.

> The Motion to be Debated is:
> That this House commends the recent announcement of a retrospective audit into surgical mesh for pelvic organ prolapse and stress urinary incontinence;
> Notes that vaginal mesh has been banned in other jurisdictions such as New Zealand;
> Further notes that NICE guidance recommends against the use of surgical mesh for pelvic organ prolapse and that no NICE recommendations have been made for stress urinary incontinence;
> Reports that Sheffield University recently announced the development of a new mesh material and calls on the Government to suspend prolapse and incontinence mesh operations while the audit is being carried out, bring forward the NICE guidelines for mesh in stress-related urinary incontinence from 2019 to 2018, and to commit to a full public inquiry into mesh if the audit suggests that this is the best course of action.

MP Emma Hardy, who led the debate, called on the government to urgently suspend all mesh implant operations. "Mesh was given to lots of young women following childbirth—many women still in their 30s—and it has left them feeling disabled. These women were injured. These women were *ignored*," she said, as members shouted "Aye!" across the historic chamber.

One of Ms. Hardy's proposals echoed a suggestion made earlier by Kath Sansom: offer physiotherapy for the pelvic floor to all new mothers as standard care by the National Health Service—as is already done in France.

What an innovative idea: help women who have just gone through vaginal childbirth start a regimen of pelvic floor–strengthening exercises to postpone prolapse and incontinence as long as possible.

In the wake of the Parliament's debate, the burden of vaginal mesh side effects on the NHS budget became the next story.

"NHS is spending hundreds of millions on care for women with vaginal mesh implants which can cause horrifying complications," read a headline in the *Independent* in April 2018.

"Health minister vows to do better" the story continued. At least £245m (roughly $315 million) had already been spent in the UK on follow-up care for women "left with debilitating, life-changing injuries." But the true cost was likely to be much higher, according to an analysis by academics at the Centre for Evidence-Based Medicine in Oxford.

Baroness Julia Cumberlege, a former health minister and member of the House of Lords went on an official tour around the country, holding meetings with women who had serious damage from mesh, preparing a report. "She is very compassionate when talking with these women," said Kath Sansom. Afterward, the Baroness Cumberlege told the press that she was "appalled at the seriousness and scale" of the damages caused by the implants.

And in July, NICE—Britain's National Institute for Health and Care Excellence—announced a moratorium on most mesh implant surgeries, in order to study the serious side effects and how to treat them.

"Yes, it was great, but you don't know what will happen next," said Kath. There's a number of doctors and surgeons in parliamentary study groups and others with influence who could affect the findings of the study.

The doctors from British medical associations fall back on research and medical articles that were funded by the mesh makers, to defend mesh, she said. "We're told surgical implants are the most studied medical devices in the world."

It's time to "take those studies apart," Kath said. The studies measure "outcomes." That measurement is "flawed!"

"What's the right outcome?" Kath said with exasperation.

The primary outcome for the sling implant is to stop incontinence. "So doctors ask their patients, 'Do you still wet your pants? No—then the implant *worked*.' They call this success," she added.

It's like measuring the success of Essure, the contraception medical device that Bayer has said it will no longer sell, after dozens of reports of serious injuries in women's reproductive organs. Kath said, "The doctors ask: 'Are you pregnant? No? That means Essure worked.' And then the women end up in hospital bleeding, needing hysterectomies."

> The primary outcome for the sling implant is to stop incontinence. "So doctors ask their patients, 'Do you still wet your pants? No—then the implant *worked*.' They call this success," she added. "The outcomes question *should be* 'Are you able to resume your normal life?'" Kath said. "That's how they should measure success."

A number of women who are members of Sling the Mesh were injured because the eroding mesh got wound around the coccyx, Kath said. They have spine issues. They can't walk. They can't sit for hours at a desk. They can't stand up to cook a meal. They're on pain medicines.

"Mesh has taken away all the joy from their lives," Kath said. One woman in 20 on her website has said she tried to commit suicide. "There's no escape from pain for them."

"The outcomes question *should be* 'Are you able to resume your normal life?'" Kath said. "That's how they should measure success."

IT'S NOT LIFE-CHANGING; IT'S LIFE-DESTROYING

Like Kath Sansom, Carolyn "Caz" Chisholm did not expect to lead a national movement to ban a medical product. She just wanted to be able to kick around a soccer ball with her son without wetting her pants.

In 2014, she underwent a procedure to implant an incontinence sling. She didn't know about problems with mesh erosion. She hadn't heard about Australia's "silent recall" of Ethicon's TVT-Secur single-incision sling in 2007.

"I was told it would be easy," said Caz. "But I had pain pretty much straight away after the surgery." She knew something was wrong with the implant, but she didn't know what it was. A Google search led her to mesh victim groups on Facebook and to Dr. Dionysios Veronikis.

Apparently, other women in Australia had serious side effects from their mesh implants. And they'd found out there were few doctors with removal surgery skills in Australia. It looked like at least 20 of them had been traveling to America for mesh revision operations with Dr. Veronikis at a hospital in St. Louis.

"I read about their injuries, and about their testimonials to him. I made an appointment and bought a plane ticket," Caz said. The removal surgery and the travel from Perth on Australia's west coast cost her some $33,000 (AUD). "I had a full removal, but I still have constant pain," she added.

She started a support group via Facebook, and soon had about 15 women communicating with her about their mesh damages. "We decided to write a letter to doctors about what we were going through." They got no response.

"'We need to hit the media,' I told them," said Caz. "I wrote to every outlet I could find. I didn't stop. I was persistent. I became a nag."

She and the group members wrote to Australia's Therapeutic Goods Administration (TGA), which oversees drugs and medical devices, like the FDA. They wrote to health ministers and deputy ministers, would-be ministers and politicians. Eventually the TGA responded. The group was put in touch with the then minister of health.

They told their stories, and several of the injured women, including Caz, were invited to Canberra to meet with TGA officials and others. The government paid for their trip to the capital in April 2016.

Caz told the director that the TGA should ban mesh. "It's not life-changing; it's life-destroying," she said. Like the US FDA, the TGA's database on adverse events in medical devices is "pretty useless."

The TGA wasn't ready to ban vaginal mesh implants, so Caz & Co. asked government officials to "at least do an ad campaign on TV" about the side effects of mesh. Some five months later, TGA put a list of adverse events connected to vaginal mesh on their website.

Caz copied that link and sent it out to other mesh support groups, and soon the 15 grew to 100. The media began paying attention, and mesh victim stories began surfacing. With that momentum, the group began pushing for an official Senate inquiry into mesh, to find out the number of women affected by mesh problems, "since the TGA wasn't going to tell us, and probably didn't know." They needed to find one or two sympathetic politicians to push for the inquiry, so they turned to Senator Derryn Hinch.

"Derryn had a track record, caring about disadvantaged people. I sent him an email late one night, and he replied in 15 minutes," Caz said. Hinch was in Melbourne on the other side of the country, and Caz jumped on a plane to meet with him.

"I didn't intend to become the advocate. It took over my life," said Caz. "But I couldn't run away."

She showed up in Melbourne with a 250-page document she had written with women's stories and medical studies she had found online, including the 2013 article by Dr. Chris Maher of Queensland called "The Transvaginal Mesh Decade." Maher wrote about the serious side effects of mesh and the need to keep conflict of interest out of medical science. He urged "arm's length" relationships between industry and doctors, having seen the effects of several mesh makers' "aggressive" marketing of their meshes in the medical community.

Caz and another mesh victim sat down with Hinch, and "he was gobsmacked." Hinch could not believe that with all the information available, mesh implants had not been banned. He agreed to send a formal letter requesting a Senate investigation into mesh.

By this time, Australian newspapers and television were digging into mesh stories. They reported on the marketing scripts used by Ethicon to recruit doctors to use mesh. And on the country's physicians' embrace of the implants. And they followed court cases in the US closer than most American media, scooping up dirt from corporate documents. But the stories with most impact involved the women across Australia whose lives had been blown apart by mesh—by the pain, by the erosion that punctured bladders and urethras and ruined sex, and by the way that doctors handled their injuries.

In February 2017, the Senate approved an inquiry and started collecting information. More than 100,000 women in Australia have had mesh implants, according to medical estimates. Many of them showed up at the public hearings on mesh that were held all across the country. Women were invited to "speak the truth," and they did. Caz said, "I heard women who said they'd told their doctors their pain wasn't from depression; it was from the implants. "No, Doctor, the mesh isn't in my head, it's in my pelvis."

> "We believe this is a catastrophic failure of the health system to protect women and ensure they have access to safe health care. We feel that women have been let down by their doctors, by the manufacturers of mesh and by the TGA (Therapeutic Goods Administration) as the regulator," the report said.

The Health Consumers' Council conducted a survey on mesh complications that showed the problem of relying on the government regulators' adverse event database. Caz said, "TGA had 99 reports. But we had 2,000 responses. What does that tell you?"

At a hearing for the review, representatives of companies like Johnson & Johnson and Boston Scientific were required to appear and answer questions. "Johnson & Johnson brought a 122-page statement with them," said Caz.

The Senate inquiry results were released in March 2018. "We believe this is a catastrophic failure of the health system to protect women and ensure they have access to safe health care. We feel that women have been let down by their doctors, by the manufacturers of mesh and by the TGA (Therapeutic Goods Administration) as the regulator," the report said.

Australian TV, radio, and newspapers reported that the Senate document showed women had been "treated appallingly" by their own physicians. And that mesh makers hadn't been transparent about the risks and complication rates of mesh implants.

> Queensland was given the OK to set up the first clinic for mesh victims. It opened in April 2019 and began scheduling patients immediately. The government is funding $3.14 million (AUD) annually.

After the Senate report was published, Australia's minister for health Greg Hunt offered a public apology to victims damaged by mesh. He promised changes and government efforts to address their suffering.

Among the Senate recommendations was an innovative medical response to the many women with serious injuries. The government was prepared to underwrite a clinic in one of the states to treat mesh victims. It would be holistic. There would be surgeons trained to remove mesh. Nurses who were experienced dealing with mesh damage. Counselors. Pain management specialists. Physiotherapists. And they would all be empathetic with the patients.

Queensland was given the OK to set up the first clinic for mesh victims. It opened in April 2019 and began scheduling patients immediately. The government is funding $3.14 million (AUD) annually.

Queensland's health minister Steven Miles said the concept of a clinic to specifically help mesh victims came from the feedback received in the Senate inquiry. "Women were going to their doctors with mesh erosion, and they weren't being believed."

"It took them organizing and vocalizing and getting to the media to break through the medical fraternity, to get them to believe women," Dr. Miles added. So government officials asked the women what they needed, and the result is "pretty unique." Queensland's Gold Coast will become recognized as the place to go to learn how to treat these women. He said, "I'm pretty proud of that."

DR. FRAZER: HE'S LISTENING

There's a little irony in the choice of the Queensland clinic's new director—Dr. Malcolm Frazer. During the 2007 "silent recall" controversy over Ethicon's TVT-Secur sling, Dr. Frazer was the source of a number of complaints to Ethicon's Aran Maree about the device and surgical failures. At the time Frazer questioned the accuracy of some of Ethicon consultants' success rates following the instructions for use, saying the directions were flawed. He told Maree he did not think that a few tweaks or tricks would improve the surgery; it needed significant changes.

"I remember that," said Dr. Frazer in an interview for this book. "The IFU was problematic, but I think the TVT-S was a problem from the beginning. We organized a two-center prospective trial, and were going to have 50 patients. We closed it down at 28 because of all the problems. In the end, we were vindicated."

The new clinic for mesh patients is an experiment in itself, said Dr. Frazer. "We began seeing patients on April 8," he exclaimed proudly.

He noted that Australia has a socialized medical system, and the clinic is only for Queensland residents or patients whose implant surgery took place in the state.

"We only accept referrals from GPs, and we triage those referrals for certain criteria," he said. "There's 'see immediately,' or 'can wait.'"

The urogynecology nurse will phone the ladies to make sure we have all their records before they are seen," he explained.

"We have a whole team," he said, adding that some are only present on certain days. "The basis of service is a multidisciplinary issue. These women's problems are not just surgical; there's issues with daily living, so there's occu therapy, and there are physiotherapists; we have chronic pain doctors, and social workers who can help the patients navigate the public health system, get the benefits of travel subsidies to come here.

"Most of the patients may need surgical intervention, and some may have already had mesh partially removed. But even then it can leave a patient with pain. Sadly, that may last forever," he added.

Frazer paused. "We had all the good intentions in the world" when vaginal mesh implants began.

"The history behind this is that we were concerned that native tissue wasn't giving us the results we wanted. There were problems with conventional repairs. So we thought maybe we shouldn't be using ordinary tissue; that may be weak."

That's how putting in a piece of artificial material to augment or replace the tissues for the lifetime of a woman became the alternative.

"But we were concerned there weren't randomized clinical trials. That there was no registry so they could be tracked and we could have real data on adverse events.

"We were unhappy with that, but we still thought mesh was a useful thing to try." In retrospect, Frazer said it was unfortunate that most of the studies were prospective and "a lot were financed by the companies themselves."

One of the first things that alarmed doctors was that with the mesh erosion, there was pain even for women sitting still. "That was a new phenomenon, and a sign that there were other things probably bubbling beneath the surface."

Frazer said one of the sadder surprises in the Senate report is the information on how doctors "ignored" their patients. "They didn't understand the pain; they didn't listen."

That's why the clinic in Queensland and others that are coming along "need to find people who are already on board with the issues.

The women need to know they wouldn't be pooh-poohed and told it was just in their heads. We don't want to make it worse for them."

FIGHTING IRISH

Commonwealth countries weren't alone in moving forward to control vaginal mesh implants. In July 2018, Ireland's government announced a pause in the use of transvaginal mesh after "understandable public anxiety." The press noted that thousands of women across the world have suffered complications after mesh implants. Ireland's Health Services would stop the use of all procedures involving transvaginal mesh devices in public hospitals. Both incontinence slings and pro-lapse kits were covered.

Ireland's Department of Health said its decision followed a review of decisions just days earlier in England and Northern Ireland to tem-porarily restrict the use of mesh until they determined how to mitigate the risks of injury to patients.

When Ireland's health officials tried to find out how many women in the country had been injured, they quickly learned that their med-ical device adverse events database was about as accurate as those of England and Australia.

That September, Ireland's "health watchdog" reported that it had not received any complaints about pelvic mesh from Irish surgeons.

Oh, it had received 76 reports about mesh-related problems.

But they were all from "the public," not doctors. In fact, more than 40 women had made presentations to Ireland's Department of Health about physical damages linked to their mesh. That group also reported difficulties accessing appropriate "aftercare" for the side effects.

The Irish surgeons' medical association responded that its mem-bers wouldn't have submitted any adverse event reports, because the rate of complications they were seeing among their patients was not higher than the expected rate, as "deduced from prior studies."

(Those would be the studies funded by the mesh makers and used by them as proof that vaginal mesh is safe and effective.)

Were all Irish women fine after mesh implants? No. Irish women had reported suffering chronic pain and recurrent infections for a number of years. Some had multiple surgeries to try to "remove" the mesh, according to a story in the *Journal* published in Dublin. Many women had to travel to the UK for the revision surgery.

"Now it has emerged that despite complications reported by women to their doctors and follow-up treatment—including surgeries—they required, not one clinician in the country notified the Health Products Regulatory Authority (HPRA)," the *Journal* of Irish news reported.

Like the US adverse event reports database at the FDA, reporting side effects to the Irish health watchdog is also voluntary. But the Irish watchdog (like the FDA) encourages doctors to report problems, because if there's a trend, early reports added together will flag it to the "signal detection" scientists at the health agency.

INDUSTRY DIGS IN

Facing an embarrassing news story about the lack of adverse events reported, surgeons who had implanted mesh turned to the president of the Continence Foundation of Ireland, Dr. Susmita Sarma, to rebuff the criticism.

The foundation's statement may sound familiar—disturbingly familiar—to mesh patients in the US and elsewhere.

"The mid-urethral sling was developed in the 1990s to treat female stress incontinence and has been extensively researched with over 2,000s papers published in this time. The known complications of mesh erosion and mesh extrusion have been well documented with a rate of 4 percent in these papers," the incontinence foundation's president said.

"Whilst reporting is encouraged by the HPRA, especially if the frequency of serious complications is above the expected reported rate, if an individual consultant was not experiencing an increased erosion rate above the expected reported rate, there would not be an indication to report same."

Dr. Sarma also said the foundation's "evidence-based" position on the use of vaginal mesh implants is that "alternative surgical treatments, which date back 60 years, are more invasive procedures" and are associated with "more complications and are less effective."

That's that. In September 2018, while British doctors were estimating complication rates swinging between 12 and 15 percent and tort lawyers in the US were pulling numbers close to 10 percent out of the confidential records of major mesh makers, gynecological doctors in Ireland were still spouting the debunked "4 percent" serious-complication or erosion rate.

> The founder of Mesh Survivors Ireland, Melanie Power (who is also a lawyer), said that most women she spoke with said that when they returned to their doctors with their complications, they got "the standard thing" from the physician: "Your problems aren't mesh related; it's the menopause." Women were also being told, "You need to break through the pain barrier." As in, "If you're having painful sex, you need to break through the pain barrier."

The founder of Mesh Survivors Ireland, Melanie Power (who is also a lawyer), said that most women she spoke with said that when they returned to their doctors with their complications, they got "the standard thing" from the physician: "Your problems aren't mesh related; it's the menopause." And that could be someone who went through the menopause 10 years beforehand, according to Ms. Power.

Women were also being told, "You need to break through the pain barrier." As in, "If you're having painful sex, you need to break through the pain barrier."

After news reports affirming serious mesh complications appeared in the press, some women spoke again to their doctors.

"They were told, 'Don't believe what you read in the media,' or 'the mesh in the news is not the mesh you have,'" according to Power's comments in the *Journal* of Irish news.

Yes, it's reasonable to wonder if a list of talking points for ob-gyns and gynecological surgeons has been e-blasted around the globe, and that is the reason all their excuses sound exactly the same.

The Irish paper's story included more context on "paternalism" by doctors in Ireland toward women patients, "verging on misogyny." But that issue, the paper reported, extended beyond the problems with vaginal mesh to other "female" conditions.

. . . US FINALLY BANS (MOST) MESH

By July 2011, when the US Food and Drug Administration published an updated warning on vaginal mesh calling serious side effects "NOT rare," its database on medical device complications was awash in notes about problems with incontinence slings and POP kits.

The FDA's report "Urogynecologic Surgical Mesh: Update on the Safety and Effectiveness of Transvaginal Placement for Pelvic Organ Prolapse" broke down the a list of nearly 4,000 adverse event reports received over the previous six years.

"The FDA conducted a search of the manufacturer and user facility device experience (MAUDE) database for medical device reports (MDRs) of adverse events associated with all urogynecologic surgical mesh products received from January 1, 2005, to December 31, 2010. The search identified 3,979 reports of injury, death, and malfunction.

"Among the 3,979 reports, 2,874 reports were received in the last 3 years (January 1, 2008–December 31, 2010), and included 1,503 reports associated with POP repairs and 1,371 associated with SUI repairs. The number of MDRs associated with POP repairs increased by more than 5-fold compared to the number of reports received in the previous 3 years (January 1, 2005–December 31, 2007)."

It's obvious that the numbers of problems reported were increasing, but even these numbers are conservative due to the problematic MAUDE database, which is a huge Achilles' heel at the FDA. According to an intensive study conducted by the International Consortium of Investigative Journalists in 2018 on medical devices, there are three major flaws involving device companies and the process of reporting to the FDA:

1. FDA inspections have found more than 4,400 violations by device companies of its rules for handling complaints and reporting device problems in the last decade. Each violation can include hundreds or even thousands of mishandled complaints.

2. Manufacturers and others required to report adverse events have classified more than 2,200 episodes in which patients died not as deaths but as *injuries,* malfunctions or other less severe events in the last five years.

3. The FDA has allowed companies such as Boston Scientific to file thousands of injury reports using a program called alternative summary reporting that allows them to keep the information from the public.

The public and media reaction to the third issue—the "alternative summary reports" that were filed in an undisclosed location (seriously)—caused the FDA to take action. In mid-2019, the agency said it was shutting down the alternative—meaning "optional"—reporting program.

Clearly, there are far too many loopholes in the approval and management of medical devices that by far benefit the pharmaceutical companies at the cost of patient health. For example, it can be a gray area to determine if the device itself caused a patient death since the body can shut down at various levels. In the case of the manufacturer Thoratec, a patient had a HeartMate II implant, which provides circulatory support to patients with advanced heart disease. When the patient died, two suspected causes of death were reported: "suspected pump thrombus," a device failure caused by a blood clot that blocks the pump, or multisystem organ failure. Thoratec's report mentions the patient's death, but cites the incident as an injury and faults organ failure as the cause of death. The obvious question here is: Did the mechanical failure cause the organs to shut down? One (of the many) problems is that with hundreds of thousands of complaints reported to the FDA's MAUDE database, it can be an insurmountable task to thoroughly evaluate each reported event. However, pump blockages were a common enough problem with this device that the FDA issued a safety warning for it in 2015.

But the fact remains that the power of the medical device industry and its lobbying behemoth AdvaMed has protected its members. The industry has waged war against efforts to close loopholes ranging from reporting deaths to conducting clinical trials for approvals.

The MAUDE database is as difficult to use as you would imagine a government website to be. Here is a list of information you need to know just to file a complaint:

- Manufacturer's name
- Product name (brand name)
- Catalog number
- Lot number
- Size
- Date of implant
- Date of explant (if mesh was removed)
- Details of the adverse event and medical and/or surgical interventions (if required)
- Reason for mesh implantation (e.g., SUI; POP)
- Type of procedure (e.g., Sling procedure: retropubic, transobturator, or mini-sling procedure for SUI; anterior repair, vaginal vault suspension, or posterior repair, for POP repair)
- Surgical approach (e.g., vaginal, abdominal, laparoscopic)
- Specific postoperative symptoms experienced by the patient with time of onset and follow-up treatment

No problem, right? Not only are the women who need to file reports struggling just to get out of bed, take care of their families, and manage their pain, but they clearly need to go to medical school in their spare time to be able to fill out this government questionnaire.

This is just one reason why we truly don't know the real devastation that mesh has caused. Most women do not know that there's a government program that collects adverse event reports, but if they try to fill out the online MAUDE questions, it's easy to get overwhelmed and discouraged.

By chance, if a patient does complete the form, their answers may vary from the next patient who has the same issues yet the results may minimize the issues. For example, one woman may say she has "stabbing pain in her vagina," while another may have been told by her doctor that the mesh eroded in her vagina, causing her this excruciating pain. Although the same issue may be in both women, the problems could be categorized separately as pain and erosion. This is yet another reason why it took so long for mesh to be banned in the US!

It took more than a decade, 100,000 lawsuits, and $8 billion to resolve patient injury claims for the US to take pelvic mesh off the market.

On April 16, 2019, the director of the FDA's Center for Devices and Radiological Health, Jeffrey Shuren, stated, "In order for these mesh devices to stay on the market, we determined that we needed evidence that they worked better than surgery without the use of mesh to repair POP. That evidence was lacking in these premarket applications, and we couldn't assure women that these devices were safe and effective in the long term.

"Patient safety is our highest priority, and women must have access to safe medical devices that provide relief from symptoms and better management of their medical conditions," he continued.

Shouldn't this have been considered *before* mesh was put on the market? Thirteen years and millions of women later, the FDA announced that "we couldn't assure women that these devices were safe and effective in the long term."

But again, this is just for situations involving pelvic organ prolapse (POP). As of May 2019, mesh is still being used for stress urinary incontinence (SUI). While POP is more prone to failure, repeat sur-geries, and injury complications, SUI still has a complication rate of approximately 5–15 percent—and a number of the women with severe, permanent injuries only got the sling. A study published in January 2018 in the journal *Female Pelvic Medicine & Reconstructive Surgery* found that "Most legal claims involved slings for SUI and began after the 2011 Food and Drug Administration communication about mesh for POP."

While banning mesh for POP was a huge step forward, there's a long way to go before American women can feel safe about medical devices that are used in and around their reproductive organs. If a doctor proposes "vaginal rejuvenation treatments," remember the mesh scandal—and run.

CHAPTER 16

REDEMPTION—A WINNING PROPOSITION

"True redemption is . . . when guilt leads to good."

—Khaled Hosseini, novelist and physician

"On behalf of the Australian government, I say sorry to all of those women with the historic agony and pain that has come from mesh implantation which have led to horrific outcomes.

"This has been an issue, over some decades in many cases, and on our time and our watch."

—Health minister of Australia Greg Hunt, October 2018

What we have seen transpire with the mesh debacle is the very essence of the worst of human nature. It is more than a cautionary tale about greed; it's a tragedy that must not be repeated.

We can't put the genie back in the bottle, but we can demand accountability. We can demand something that resembles redemption. There is no way that this mass litigation can end with medical device makers, doctors, and lawyers being able to keep millions of dollars (hundreds of millions for some) in their pockets. We also can't walk away, and let the FDA maintain the status quo, by forgoing how medical devices are registered and mass-marketed.

The system is broken. But there are realistic ways that it can be fixed:

- Women with severe injuries must receive appropriate medical treatment, including mesh removal surgery if necessary.
- The mesh maker corporations, the doctors' specialty medical associations that promoted mesh implants, and lawyers who received tens of millions of dollars in administrative fees in the multidistrict litigation should all contribute to this medical rehab program.
- The program should include creation of multiple mesh medical centers around the country, and training in mesh removal surgery. Australia already has such centers for integrated treatment—surgery, pain management, counseling for women who can no longer have sex, and physical therapy.
- From now on, there must be registries for any implants, including mesh, with details on the model and the date of surgery. Implant registries, which mesh makers have tried to stop, should provide the kind of information and details that we demand from automakers about all the parts in our cars.
- The overused and abused 510(k) approval process must be fixed. It's abusive and criminal. And it has produced too many medical product disasters. The Food and Drug Administration must stand up to the medical device industry and its Washington, DC, lobbying group AdvaMed.
- The mass tort system failed mesh victims. For mesh it demonstrated that the standard mass tort–MDL process only served the defendant corporations, their attorneys, and the mass tort lawyers. It is time to develop a different way to deal with major product liability litigation that involves thousands or more plaintiffs with damages. And nobody should be off the hook here.

MEDICAL DEVICE MAKERS

Medical device makers need to adjust their sights to promote patient health rather than solely conjuring up profits. But that's unlikely to happen soon.

So here's a unique approach: when patients are injured by products that were meant to help them, these corporations should be required to pay for the patients' repair surgeries and treatments.

Let's pretend that we could rewind time and rewrite history.

Imagine that it's 1998 and ProteGen is about to be OK'd for sale in America; the Boston Scientific marketing team is planning its strategy. If Boston Scientific knew that it had to pay for every instance of erosion, migration, infection, and more, would they have pushed it so hard to doctors? Would 17,000 women have been implanted with an untested product if Boston Scientific knew that they would be billed by hospitals for every removal surgery, ER visit, pain and antibiotic prescription—perhaps even for lost wages due each patient?

Let's also add that these financial payments would be separate from settlements and beyond punitive and compensatory damages.

Medical device companies need to be held responsible for the damages they've caused. Women whose vaginas were destroyed due to mesh implants need the option to go to surgery centers funded by the companies who made the dangerous products, so they can get the medical help they so desperately need. The humane action would be for these device makers to create these centers across the US, using the profits they made off these patients.

(Note to mesh makers: Another country, one with far less money than America, has already started such medical centers for vaginal mesh victims. Hint: Down Under.)

Funding and conducting *impartial* medical studies that are accurate, thorough, involve a minimum number of patients, and are followed for several years is another way to stop faulty products from being put on the market.

Think back to how vaginal mesh was "studied." Ulf Ulmsten was propositioned by Johnson & Johnson that if he reported high success rates, he would be paid $1 million. This resulted in carnage; imagine what the outcome could have been in the wake of an unbiased report.

Mesh makers still don't want to admit their implants were inherently dangerous. For example, a former AMS executive is trying to get two of these mesh implants back on the market. John Nealon, who launched a new medical device company of his own in 2018 called UroCure, feels that this is the right time to relaunch AMS vaginal implants based on the SPARC and other models for patient use (and note that there are approximately 22,000 lawsuits filed against these AMS products).

If you're interested in knowing what John Nealon's roles were at AMS, his titles included vice president of global marketing, senior vice president of business development, and senior vice president and general manager for AMS Women's Health—elevated company positions. But even after so many countries have banned the use of vaginal mesh and with all the information about mesh risks now public—thanks to lawsuits—Mr. Nealon is prepared to embrace another vaginal mesh company. In 2019, UroCure sponsored a booth at the annual American Urological Association convention, held in Chicago. It said: "UroCure—Advancing Women's Health." And it promoted the ArcTV Transvaginal Sling System.

Perhaps there should be greater, or even criminal, penalties to hold corporate *executives* accountable so that they'll calculate the cost of patient lives and not just calculate their profits.

Device makers made billions of dollars from mesh at the expense of every woman and family out there. They may have paid out chunks of settlements for irreparable damage, but per person these unmeaningful settlements amounted to approximately $3,000 to $150,000—and the average was about $60,000.

Then you deduct 40 percent legal fees, 5 percent MDL fees, "expenses" that the law firm determines unilaterally and add on existing medical liens—and many women actually end up owing money. There is no money to cover any more medical bills required to repair damages. And, of course, it doesn't begin to cover lost income or the pain, suffering, broken relationships, and more that have devastated these women.

Look at the numbers—some two million women had mesh implants in the US—either incontinence slings or prolapse supports. We know that "complication rates" are much higher than the 4 or 5 percent reported by mesh makers in their funded research. The United Kingdom's National Health System has estimated complications among up to 15 percent of patients.

Even at 10 percent, that means roughly 200,000 women need—or will need—surgery to remove mesh or repair serious erosions, fix perforations to organs such as the bladder and urethra. And even if patients believe their implants are fine now, remember that Drs. Margolis, Veronikis, Garely, and Raz all say that they have treated mesh victims whose procedures had been performed years earlier—even up to 10 years. Polypropylene mesh doesn't respond to deadlines; it can wait you out.

So what would 200,000 removal surgeries cost our health system? How many women who have undergone "revision" or removal surgery require multiple operations? By now, you've probably read about women in their 40s and 50s who have faced five or more mesh-related surgeries. Add to the cost of these surgeries the many ER visits, prescription medications, and the misdiagnosis of pain that so many women have undergone, and you'll quickly see that this mesh tragedy is not only a colossal problem that these women have to maneuver through but also a huge burden on the health-care system.

And who will pay? Third-party insurers? Medicare and Medicaid? The women and their families? Haven't they paid enough?

This is why a mesh treatment center is a necessary and good investment. Imagine if we combined the funds being paid for reconstructive surgeries and the related treatment options and put them into specialized facilities to get real help for these women. Pay experts to train other doctors in removal techniques. Cover the costs of scans and ultrasounds, bladder tests and blood tests—set test-result standards related to what we already know about mesh damage.

Include pain management experts, too. After all, many women who had successful removal operations are still in terrible pain because of the permanent damage done by the eroding, shrinking, or clinging mesh. As Dr. Margolis says, "Sometimes I have to tell a patient there is nothing more I can do to help her. But that doesn't mean all her injuries have been repaired, just that there's no safe way to perform further surgery."

Bring in counselors and psychologists, family therapists who can talk with couples about their inability to have intercourse because of mesh complications. Get physical therapists. Hire nurses and physicians who actually have seen mesh patients unable to walk because of nerve damage. The corporations can afford to do this.

THE DOCTORS

Doctors have eroded the very fabric of the trust between a physician and his patients with mesh. What happened to their "Do No Harm" code? Mesh doctors did harm, and they did it for money.

In fact, they are still doing it. At the time of this book's publication, POP kits have been withdrawn in the US—either voluntarily or at the direction of the FDA. But some urologists and ob-gyns are still putting in versions of POP kit mesh for prolapse. And a number of ob-gyns are still implanting mesh incontinence slings.

One of the seriously injured women interviewed for this book was just told by her own doctor that she, the doctor, is still doing mesh implants. The doctor told her patient that just a "few" women had complications—a nice version of "suffered severe side effects," and that studies show it's "safe." "I didn't know what to say to my doctor, I was so shocked," the woman said.

Doctors must help these women get back on their feet by helping to treat them into the future.

Most of these doctors we know, from the people who "trained" them in mesh, were in fact under-trained. Most of them weren't urologists. Still, they had the arrogance to think that they could perform such a delicate procedure after one training session. They should give their time to resolve the injuries they caused.

Currently too many women are living with mesh complications and too few doctors know how to remove it. Many women are using their own bank accounts to pay for flights across the nation and even across the world to meet with specialists. The doctors who did multiple implants could attend seminars on how to remove the entangled mesh from experts and then donate their hours in surgery centers to repair what they've destroyed.

Some doctors are boasting that they can remove mesh all the while they're just cutting the loose pieces out. Many times, partial removals do more harm than good because these doctors aren't properly trained. But doctors never want to admit that. Training is key; hence, certified mesh surgical centers would give women the confidence and relief to manage their TVM complications.

Doctors' elite medical associations like ACOG (American College of Obstetricians and Gynecologists) and AUGS (American Urogynecologic Society) were complicit in the mesh disaster. They carried the message of the corporations to their members, and did the companies' marketing for them. Those professional organizations should repay some of the damage they allowed, by funding training programs for mesh removal in their district groups.

The organizations should also make their members attend more courses that detail ways to treat some of the other injuries related to mesh erosion. For example, women who have serious mesh erosion in their pelvic area have chronic UTIs—urinary tract infections. But in hundreds of mesh cases in the MDL and in the states, women said their ob-gyns didn't treat them with antibiotics. Instead, their doctors ignored the symptoms—burning during urination and pain—until many of these women ended up at emergency rooms (where doctors on call took a quick list of the symptoms, did an exam, read that the patient had had a vaginal mesh implant, and connected the dots on the spot).

Ob-gyns and urogynecologists should know about the many side effects of eroded mesh implants by now; there is no excuse for failing to treat obvious conditions like repeated UTIs. These medical groups should ensure that their members know the various problems associated with mesh erosion—or where to call for help. There are other, safer ways to solve stress urinary incontinence and pelvic organ prolapse.

Physicians should learn from the mesh debacle. Before using any drug or device, doctors need to research what they're putting into their patients' bodies and look beyond the device maker rep's sales pitch. They should research independent studies, or even wait until the product has been on the market for several years to ensure its safety. They should realize that newer isn't always best.

THE FDA

The 510(k) loophole doesn't work; in fact, it's putting millions of people's lives and health at risk with minimal product testing, lack of methods to track and monitor drugs and medical devices, and no help for patients when they experience harsh adverse effects. Innovation without accountability causes the masses to become the silent guinea pigs and lab rats who are used and tossed aside all in the name of "progress." In this day and age, we should be worth more than that.

After all the studies and device controversies presented to the FDA, would the members of this government organization want vaginal mesh inserted into their bodies or the vaginas of their wives or daughters? Why did they let this genital mutilation destroy thousands of American women's lives for two decades?

> Former FDA commissioner Dr. David Kessler said, "The system we set up does not work." In an interview for this book, Kessler noted that even physicians do not realize how most medical devices are approved for sale by the FDA, and how little clinical data there is on many devices' safety and efficacy.

Former FDA commissioner Dr. David Kessler said, "The system we set up does not work." In an interview for this book, Kessler noted that even physicians do not realize how most medical devices are approved for sale by the FDA, and how little clinical data there is on many devices' safety and efficacy. "Even with everything on the news about medical device problems, doctors really do not understand the regulation of medical devices and implants. Doctors make assumptions like the average American" that a special medical body carefully studied the device before approving it for sale.

Dr. Adriane Fugh-Berman, professor of pharmacology and physiology at Georgetown University, also interviewed for *The Bleeding Edge*, said she and her colleagues have been surprised to see how little surgeons know about medical device standards. "Some of the surgeons seemed to think that, 'well, the FDA had taken care of this, that of course these devices had been tested in humans.'"

Today, it's estimated that 32 million Americans have at least one medical device. Last year an investigative series by a journalism consortium that included the Associated Press found that about 1.7 million injuries and 80,000 deaths have been linked to medical devices over the past decade.

The 510(k) process was enacted in 1976. Why are we still maintaining an antiquated system for something as important and potentially dangerous as the medical devices that we put inside our bodies?

The 510(k) pass must be stopped. "That provision is a loophole. It was meant as an exception. But that exception is now the rule," Dr. Kessler says.

Furthermore, if a product has been recalled, it should not become the basis (a.k.a. "substantially equivalent") for a new product to be fast-tracked to market. Clearly, there was something terribly wrong with the product, so why in the world would we want another mistaken device put in its place?

If this logical concept had been enacted when ProteGen was recalled, hundreds of thousands of women could have been spared the agony of mesh. And it didn't matter that the pore size, thread size, or insertion tools changed; it all contained plastic mesh that erodes in the body. It's like putting arsenic in a variety of cocktails. Changing the other ingredients won't change the outcome.

"I called the FDA and asked them, 'How can you clear something based on a predicate device that's already been shown to be dangerous?'" said health-care writer Jeanne Lenzer during *The Bleeding Edge* documentary. The FDA told her, "We don't judge what the prior device is." Lenzer is the author of the *Danger Within Us*, about the flawed medical devices and FDA 510(k) clearance process.

"So even if the device was recalled because it was dangerous," explains Dr. Rita Redberg, editor of the *Journal of the American Medical Association's Internal Medicine*, "you can still use it as a predicate and get your device cleared" because it's considered "substantially equivalent."

IT'S TIME TO BUILD A REGISTRY

"The FDA is sometimes kept in the dark by medical device makers. We just assume the FDA has the data that they need to crack down on manufacturers that have bad devices. We think they have real-time information that allows them to recall a product. But the FDA does not have that," said Madris Tomes, former FDA analyst and now CEO of Device Events, in an interview for this book. She was originally brought in by the FDA to help "fix" its muddled adverse event reporting system called MAUDE. "It was almost unmanageable, and companies found many ways to avoid full disclosure using that system," Tomes said.

This is why the FDA needs to create a registry that tracks and monitors what exact medical device a patient has (brand, model, serial number), the surgeon's name who implanted it, and for what condition it was intended to fix. Think that this is too expensive or complicated to pursue?

That's what industry says. Mesh makers have been reluctant to create mesh registries. The attorney general of California, which is suing Johnson & Johnson over mesh damages, found out why.

J&J HID KNOWN MESH RISKS DUE TO COMPETITIVE DISADVANTAGE

From an Exhibit by Plaintiffs in State of California v Johnson & Johnson trial 2019.	"When any adverse event is captured in a registry, it has to be reported... Consequently, if none of our competitors are keeping registries, our complications data may appear increasingly accurate but with decreasing appeal" - *Dr. David Robinson, J&J Medical Director*

(This is a slide from the AG's office shown in court during the trial of *State of California v. Ethicon et al.* in July 2019.)

> If you have a mesh registry, it has to pick up any adverse events. That's data, and too much data on complications, as you can read, might cause doctors and patients to avoid the implant.

Yes, there it is in an email from one of Johnson & Johnson's medical directors, David Robinson: If you have a mesh registry, it has to pick up any adverse events. That's data, and too much data on complications, as you can read, might cause doctors and patients to avoid the implant.

Industry has been able to play with the FDA's medical device adverse events reporting system, MAUDE—even getting permission to roll hundreds of reports of complications into a single event filing, and even then, not releasing it to the public. Registries, even retrospective registries, would change that.

Consider the automotive industry. There have been many recalls in recent years involving Takata airbags, hydraulic brakes, rear suspension systems, and more, and it's highly likely that you've received a notification from your dealership or car manufacturer to address the problem. Additionally, they recommend that you bring your car in immediately so that they can fix the problem—for FREE. They acknowledge it was their mistake.

We demand this for our cars, trucks, and minivans, but we accept malfunctioning parts that go inside of our bodies, all the while eating the high costs of medical bills and never getting a word of apology or warning from the medical device company.

Without a notice from the company, the only way that we know an implant is faulty is because we're having problems with it, our doctor mentions it to us, or we see ads on TV or the internet from law firms recruiting clients to sue the maker—and by then it could be too late to fix. Imagine what a registry and printed cards that inform caregivers about the patient's implant could do to ease patients' medical problems. No second-guessing. No wasted treatments. No multiple doctor or hospital visits. Just the direct care needed to help a patient in crisis.

Australia has created device-specific registries due to their similar health complications involving pelvic mesh, hip replacements, cardiac devices, and breast implants. The nation is considering creating a national registry to monitor all devices.

Opponents argue that maintaining a system this large for an undetermined length of time is too expensive, but ABC News Australia's rebuttal is simple: "This cost would be offset by the cost to the health system of patients with defective devices not being detected . . . Given the speed with which medical technology is advancing, the industry and the government cannot afford to ignore this issue."

A medical registry would prevent and solve so many basic problems. Hospital records are great, but they don't track medical devices in a way that is valuable to the patient. Furthermore, as many women with mesh learned when they signed up for lawsuits, some hospital records simply disappear. Who knows why.

But a registry would track if, when, and what treatment a patient had and would help to diagnose problems more accurately down the line. Consider that many women never even knew they had mesh and only found out after experiencing horrible ailments and visiting multiple doctors. A registry could have helped these women much earlier in the process or even eliminated most of these problems, because a cohesive record of mesh complications would have been in place. It only makes sense to track a device that is implanted in the body.

Doctors aren't required to report adverse events, only medical device companies are, but would they really share the dangers of their products at the risk of reducing profits? Obviously not. The mesh files have company documents and emails showing how some mesh makers chose to "identify" complications with their implants as "not" unusual. This negligence of reporting allows devices to be on the market for longer than they should be, allowing for thousands of patients to be put at risk. This has to stop!

If women knew what kind of surgical mesh they had or that mesh was the culprit for their pain, bleeding, or various debilitating autoimmune symptoms for conditions like lupus, they could have kept their insurance and jobs—which seems like pure luxury now.

They could have received treatment and not been denied the truth, told "it's all in your head," or belittled. In fact, as we were concluding this book, we received this email from Robin B. who was so frustrated by her most recent appointment with a new doctor:

> The new primary care doctor humiliated me, he said he wanted to do a physical. Well, he didn't take my blood or urine, he wanted to take a pap smear, I said "no" when I saw a large speculum and questioned his testing a neovagina. He listened to my heart and lungs, then wanted to look at my genitals. He made a comment that I didn't look mutilated!! Which my husband spoke up and said my problems were internal. I was so upset, felt on display. I felt disgusted that he wanted just to look. Curiosity, with no professionalism. It felt like emotional rape . . .
>
> I received no real treatment and now today I took pictures—my neovagina/bladder is coming out of me

. . . If I could change my scenario, I would. I must be a target for medical abuse. I really want it to quit!

THE LAWYERS

Lawyers on various committees for the national multidistrict litigation—the MDL—were awarded more than half a billion dollars for their "leadership" fee, which they split among themselves. That amount is in addition to the roughly 40 percent fees for each client who settled, and reimbursement for expenses. A portion of this $500 million could set up treatment centers all over the US to help these women who need revision and/or removal surgeries and pain management therapies.

But this isn't some cry for so-called tort reform. It's quite the opposite. Tort reform just further limits consumers' rights that have already been eroded by corporate-funded attacks on lawsuits, like the campaign by the national Chamber of Commerce. Tort reform is a slippery slope designed to cut off all chances for victims of product liability to seek compensation for their injuries.

But too many big-name lawyers who vowed to help mesh victims have accumulated fortunes, while the women they were hired to help are abandoned, broke, and devastated. Hiring lawyers is one of the only ways consumers can get help using a system that would otherwise be inaccessible to them. It's time that lawyers accept their responsibility for turning the mesh MDL into a lawyers' feeding frenzy.

Judge Joseph Goodwin of the MDL should withdraw the leadership fee he has approved, and instead mandate that part of it—say, 20 percent?—go into a fund to help women pay for treatment and surgeries, toward improving their quality of life.

A tort attorney, who's a player in what is colloquially called the "Houston Mafia," made a crude comment a couple of years ago about the benefits of the vaginal mesh craze. He said lawyers would make a fortune off the "holocaust of pussy." (More on that later.)

He was right—he and others have made literally hundreds of millions of dollars by skimming off the vast number of women who got screwed in this disaster.

Multidistrict litigations (MDLs) need serious reform, too. They were created to make sure the system wasn't too inundated and that consumers got swift justice, but now they're just a playground for grown-up fraternity boys who get out of law school and have no idea what it's like to take a deposition or work up a case. The lawyers who've been doing this for a long while are the same players, with the same judges, appointing the same people to oversee the litigations at private residences and on private planes all over the world. It's not only cozy but incestuous.

The same 20 firms should not automatically turn up on every leadership committee, appointing their friends to subcommittees to "oversee fees" on vaginal mesh, 3M, and other ligation that's coming down the pipeline.

FOLLOW THE LEADER

Australia has been light-years ahead of the United States when it comes to taking TVM off the market and addressing the resulting problems of women. Their Department of Health Therapeutic Goods Administration (TGA) officially banned mesh use for pelvic organ prolapse on November 28, 2017 (almost a year and a half before the US recalled POP kits), and thereafter has been building an infrastructure to help women devastated by vaginal mesh. The Australian government has taken the following steps, and it would be wise for our government to follow suit.

ISSUED AN APOLOGY

In October 2018, Health Minister Greg Hunt presented a heartfelt speech and commented: "On behalf of the Australian government, I say sorry to all of those women with the historic agony and pain that has come from mesh implantation which have led to horrific outcomes.

"This has been an issue, over some decades in many cases, and on our time and our watch."

> "On behalf of the Australian government, I say sorry to all of those women with the historic agony and pain that has come from mesh implantation which have led to horrific outcomes. "This has been an issue, over some decades in many cases, and on our time and our watch."

GOT THE WORD OUT THAT MESH IS HARMFUL

In Australia's Medicare Benefits Schedule Review Taskforce report from the Gynaecology Clinical Committee of 2018, Section 6 states:

> After a review of the clinical evidence, the TGA found that the benefits of using transvaginal mesh products in the treatment of pelvic organ prolapse do not out-weigh the risks these products pose to patients.
>
> In independently reviewing the evidence, the Committee identified problems with MBS items involving the use of mesh and developed recommen-dations to address patient safety. Following the TGA's announcement regarding regulatory actions in rela-tion to transvaginal mesh products and single-incision mini-slings, the Committee revised its recommenda-tions to align with the TGA, and as a result there will be no MBS items available that will allow for the use of graft (mesh) material in the treatment of pelvic organ prolapse.

Acknowledging the problem is one thing; addressing it is another. Fortunately, this is an important item on Australia's agenda.

The faculty of medicine from the University of Queensland announced on June 7, 2017, that "those affected by ongoing complications associated with transvaginal mesh can be reassured Australian specialists are leaders in the management of these problems. Not only were we among the first in the world to report large trials that evaluated transvaginal mesh, we've also reported on the safety, technique and efficacy of mesh-removal procedures for vaginal pain in peer-reviewed publications."

CONDUCTED A SENATE INQUIRY

The Parliament of Australia conducted a year-long inquiry researching the causes and the extent of damages created by the mesh debacle. In a report published on March 28, 2018, they created a plan to prevent another large-scale medical device tragedy from devastating their country again.

> "Women that have had those implants, who have those outcomes . . . have been failed in a monumental way by the system and by certain people in the medical profession who they trusted," said Senator Rachel Siewert when she introduced the report to the Senate. "I hope that we never have to have another inquiry where we see such suffering from the witnesses."

The report addressed crucial recommendations for improved treatment guidelines and medical training, prevention of financial kickbacks for doctors, a registry of high-risk implantable devices, and an audit of past procedures. It also cited concern that accurately identifying the number of women who have already received TVM implants in the country is impossible, so a registry is vital to consumer health.

"Women that have had those implants, who have those outcomes . . . have been failed in a monumental way by the system and by certain people in the medical profession who they trusted," said Senator Rachel Siewert when she introduced the report to the Senate. "I hope that we never have to have another inquiry where we see such suffering from the witnesses."

"I hope our report convinces them they have been listened to and more importantly they have been believed," Senator Derryn Hinch said at the Senate meeting as he introduced the report.

"It was very clear in the report that women who have experienced adverse complications as a result of a mesh implant have endured long-term pain and reduced quality of life," said Professor Steve Robson from the Royal Australian and New Zealand College of Obstetricians and Gynaecologists, which trains and accredits doctors in Australia and New Zealand.

POLITICAL ACTION

This causes us to wonder, where have the US politicians been? Why have they been missing for years? Women's rights and health-care issues are hot topics, and yet this one keeps getting swept under the rug. It's time for our elected officials to step up and protect the very women who are voting for them.

Kamala Harris, in May 2016, filed a lawsuit as California attorney general against Johnson & Johnson. She said she was fighting against companies' alleged false advertising and deceptive marketing of their surgical mesh products for women. "Johnson & Johnson put millions of women at risk of severe health problems by failing to provide critical information to doctors and patients about its surgical mesh products," her office stated. What happened to the passion for this issue?

Senator Harris, Vice President Joe Biden, Representative Jackie Speier, and Donald Trump—where are you? You can't address the health-care cost crisis if you don't address issues like mesh that are costing so much.

BEGAN MESH REMOVAL CENTERS

The Royal Australian and New Zealand College of Obstetricians and Gynaecologists (RANZCOG) had specifically addressed the need for trained doctors and surgery centers dedicated to the removal of vaginal mesh. They have published a "mesh removal information sheet" that not only apologizes for the complications that women are having due to mesh but also helps them to find surgery centers near them with teams of doctors to provide a cohesive plan for recovery. This sheet explains that

> Every woman's clinical situation is different, and it is important to understand that mesh removal surgery may not address all of the symptoms that a woman may be experiencing. For this reason, mesh removal may not be an appropriate option. However, overall, we advise the factors that are important for women who may be considering a mesh removal procedure to understand are:
> - the unit where the removal surgery is planned should have experience in mesh removal;
> - ideally, mesh removal should be carried out as part of a multidisciplinary unit with access to a urologist, colorectal surgeon and/or pain specialist, and a specialist pelvic floor physiotherapist.
>
> RANZCOG recommends that women who are seeking guidance on mesh removal specialists in Australia and New Zealand seek assistance from a unit with a urogynaecologist. RANZCOG is able to confirm that this group of specialists has received formal training in mesh removal as part of their training Fellowship.

The Queensland Pelvic Mesh Service has even been set in place and is composed of "a team of medical, nursing and allied health specialists, offering expertise in surgery, continence care, chronic pain management and counseling."

"There are many women who are experiencing significant health problems caused by pelvic mesh devices," Steven Miles, the minister for health, said. "We are committed to providing specialised care and treatment for women, whether they live in rural, remote, regional or metropolitan Queensland.

"This highly specialised interdisciplinary service will be delivered on the Gold Coast, meaning all the expertise in caring for and treating women with pelvic mesh complications is available at the one site.

"Due to the complexity of mesh complications, each woman will have very different needs."

Australia is setting up "interdisciplinary" centers to treat mesh victims. "The Queensland Pelvic Mesh Service will include an initial comprehensive interdisciplinary assessment, resulting in a plan of care developed with each woman to meet her needs, including her recovery goals."

Department of Health

Media Statement

Queensland
Government

---

xx December 2019

Gold Coast to host service dedicated to women affected by pelvic mesh

A specialized service for women with pelvic mesh complications is expected to open on the Gold Coast in the first half of 2019.

The Queensland Pelvic Mesh Service will comprise a team of medical, nursing and allied health specialists, offering expertise in surgery, continence care, chronic pain management and counseling.

The service has been co-designed with clinicians, Health Consumers Queensland and consumer representatives to ensure it will meet the needs of affected women.

"There are many women who are experiencing significant health problems caused by pelvic mesh devices, " Minister for Health and Ambulance Services, Steven Miles said.

"We are committed to providing specialized care and treatment for women, whether they live in rural, remote, regional or metropolitan Queensland.

"This highly specialized interdisciplinary service will be delivered on the Gold Coast, meaning all the expertise in caring for and treating women with pelvic mesh complications is available at the one site."

"Due to its complexity of mesh complications, each woman will have different needs."

"The Queensland Pelvic Mesh Service will include an initial comprehension interdisciplinary assessment, resulting in a plan of care developed with each woman to meet her needs, including her recovery goals."

Minister Miles said women across the state will have equitable access to the service, which will offer a range of treatments, procedures and support.

He said the Queensland Health Patient Travel Subsidy Scheme will subside travel and accommodation costs for eligible women.

"Based on the interdisciplinary assessment and in consultation with women, care and treatment will be offered relevant to recovery needs," he said.

"This care may include medical and nursing treatment and procedures, continence care, chronic pain management, counseling, psychology, social work support and physiotherapy."

In 2018, the Therapeutic Goods Administration (TGA) restricted the sale of transvaginal mesh products designed by solely for the treatment of pelvic organ prolapse and single incision mini-slings used to treat stress urinary incontinence.

The action was taken after a TGA review determined the risks of using transvaginal mesh for pelvic organ prolapse outweighed urinary incontinence.

Queensland's center gets government funding, which is about $3.14 million annually. But then, Australia doesn't have anywhere near the number of mesh patients as we have in the US.

What could American medical programs do with $100 million—that is, 20 percent of the MDL leadership committee fees. It's pennies in the $8 billion in legal costs and settlements to mesh makers. Why can't we set up statewide or regional mesh treatment centers . . . or both? If Australia can do it, certainly the US can, too, especially since this blueprint has already been created!

WHAT CAN PATIENTS DO?

- Research any device that a doctor or surgeon recommends should be used in you.
- Don't feel embarrassed to get a second option/opinion.
- Newer isn't always better.
- Ask your surgeon how many of these procedures he or she has performed.
- To see if your doctor has been paid by a medical device company, go to openpaymentsdata.cms.gov.
- Keep a copy of all current medical records from doctor's visits to medications, to diagnostic testing.
- Don't be embarrassed to ask any questions. You're your best advocate.
- Not sure what to ask your doctor? Get online and on Facebook and find groups like Mesh Victims United, whose members can give you advice and tell you how they tackled their damage.
- Finally, write your representative in Congress and your senators if you've been injured—let them know you want to be counted, and you want accountability.
- Demand hearings on mesh failures in Congress and in statehouses—shed some light on what these companies and these medical associations did because of greed.
- Remember: you are *not* alone.

We can't put the genie back in the bottle, but we can't just move on from mesh like the doctors and lawyers who say they have "mesh fatigue." The mesh victims can't just move on. Medical devices like mesh have evolved from a cautionary tale into a modern-day tragedy. This should never happen again.

TVM TIMELINE OF DESTRUCTION

Now this whole story contains a lot of information to take in, so here's a snapshot of some of the main points. This is an outrageous debacle, and the women involved should be outraged that in 1999 ProteGen was recalled, but mesh wasn't banned in the US until 2019. Or why was mesh cleared for pelvic organ prolapse just one year *after* French scientists published a report on the complications involved with mesh? If so many women started going to their doctors because their mesh was eroding and migrating, why weren't more doctors trained and research done to help these women? The more you look at this timeline, the more this tragedy just doesn't make sense.

1951—Polypropylene is invented.

1958—Polypropylene is applied to surgical procedures.

1976—The FDA adopts the 510(k) process to fast-track medical devices to market.

1987—Polypropylene mesh is commonly used in hernia repair surgeries.

1996—Ulf Ulmsten publishes a paper explaining his new method of using polypropylene mesh to repair stress urinary incontinence (SUI).

ProteGen Sling is cleared by the FDA through 510(k) process.

1997—ProteGen Sling enters the market. In just two months, Boston Scientific sold almost $1 million worth of the slings.

1998—Boston Scientific memo reveals that "in hindsight, to launch ProteGen, [Boston Scientific] needed greater understanding of ProteGen risks." They knew that there was a 5 percent complication rate, 18 percent of doctors who used it were dissatisfied with the product, and one-third of doctors who used it planned to never use it again. The most common complication was erosion resulting in damage to sliced urethras and bladders.

In June, the FDA visits Boston Scientific and learns that two-thirds of the complications that are reported to the company concern the vaginal slings. They *still* determine that there is no need for a recall.

1999—In January, Boston Scientific announces it will **recall ProteGen** after 17,000 women have been implanted with the device.

2001—Vaginal mesh "kits" hit the market for greater appeal to doctors.

2003—French scientist and mesh expert Dr. Cosson writes to Ethicon, saying Johnson & Johnson's Prolift had problems with the mesh material, including erosion (exposure through the vaginal wall or into organs), contraction (scar tissue around the mesh pushes it together), and recurrence (the return of prolapse).

2004—FDA clears pelvic mesh for conditions involving pelvic organ prolapse (POP).

2005—In March, Prolift enters the market without FDA approval. Around that same time, Dr. Cosson publishes study findings involving the Prolift mesh. He and his team found that of the 277 patients in the study, 34 women had experienced mesh exposure. After a month of treatment, 25 required surgery.

Chevron Phillips refuses to be Boston Scientific's supply of Marlex due to the controversy over plastics in the body and stated, "We are simply not interested in this business at any price."

2007—TVT-Secur is reported to have a 30 percent failure rate.

TVT-experienced doctors in Australia were seeing "failure" rates of 25–50 percent.

In November, Johnson & Johnson's director of safety for medical devices in Australia and New Zealand, Aran Maree, bagins a silent recall of TVT-Secur in Australia, **but TVT-Secur is still used in the US.**

2008—FDA published the first alert pertaining to vaginal mesh complications.

2009—Approximately 2,000 women each month get some type of POP implant.

2010—The first mesh claims are consolidated into multidistrict litigation cases in West Virginia.

2011—Dr. Michael Thomas Margolis testifies before an FDA advisory panel in September explaining that "it is difficult if not impossible to remove all the mesh and do it safely."

The FDA finally acknowledges that "serious adverse events are NOT rare" concerning TVM and publishes a safety communication in July. In September, most manufacturers elected to stop marketing surgical mesh for transvaginal repair of POP after the FDA requires these companies to conduct postmarket surveillance studies.

2012—Prolift removed from market "for business reasons" two years *after* a patient dies from complications due to Prolift surgery.

Boston Scientific is accused of using forfeit Chinese plastics in their mesh products.

2013—A study followed 58 women who required mesh removal surgery: of those 17 (29 percent) required an additional surgery to remove the residual mesh, 13 of them once and 4 twice.

2016—The FDA changed vaginal mesh from being a Class II device (moderate risk) to a Class III (high risk).

2017—New Zealand bans vaginal mesh for POP.

2018—It's estimated that between three to four million women have vaginal mesh worldwide. Of those women, 150,000 to 200,000 experience severe complications.

Australia bans pelvic mesh for POP in January.

Ireland bans pelvic mesh for SUI in July.

UK bans pelvic mesh for POP in December.

2019—In March, the FDA announces that they are looking deeper into the link between medical devices and autoimmune disorders.

The US bans pelvic mesh for POP in April, **20 years** after the first recall.

SOURCES

I relied largely on documents, PowerPoint sets, and emails from Johnson & Johnson, Boston Scientific, and American Medical Systems obtained through the multidistrict litigation (MDL) on vaginal mesh.

Those documents, which dated back to the 1980s, were only the skeleton. Other materials included the transcripts of multiple meetings at the FDA regarding vaginal mesh in 2011 and 2019, as well as interviews with many current and former officials at the FDA and its Center for Devices and Radiological Health (CDRH).

I reviewed the FDA document packages prepared for 2011 and 2019 public hearings; position statements from AdvaMed, lobbyists for the medical device industry; and correspondence between the FDA and AdvaMed members on mesh. Other documents reviewed:

- The 2009 FDA report from CDRH on the Menaflex knee device mesh clearance
- The Institute of Medicine 2001 report on the FDA's 510(k) process for device clearance
- GAO reports on FDA medical device issues including clearances and PMA approvals

The report of the Australian Senate in 2018 was invaluable.

I've read position statements from AUGS and ACOG on transvaginal mesh and their communications with the FDA and statements for FDA advisory committee hearings in 2011 and 2019. I studied the Scientific Committee on Emerging and Newly Identified Health

Risks 2015 opinion on the safety of surgical meshes used in urogyne-cological surgery.

Transcripts of seven trials involving vaginal mesh were also read and consulted. There were transcripts and videos of depositions of leading corporate figures involved in mesh marketing and development decisions. And I watched a number of days of live trials on Courtroom View Network.

I reviewed exhibits from those trials. I saw many documents from lawyers in the MDL including work products.

Detailed investigations into mesh by the *Guardian* in the UK, the *Daily Mail*, the *British Medical Journal*, and ABC News in Australia were invaluable.

Another important resource was the nearly daily report from Jane Akre of the Mesh Medical Device News Desk.

I interviewed over 20 doctors who implant mesh, remove it, or both, from the US, France, UK, Australia, New Zealand, Israel, and Sweden.

There were interviews with nurses and nurse practitioners. I attended the AUGS conference for Pelvic Floor Disorders Week in Chicago after I formally obtained a press pass, but I was not allowed into any of the scientific sessions or meetings and was followed by communications staff for AUGS.

Two dozen lawyers for plaintiffs and one brave lawyer for a mesh maker talked with me.

Some 45 women allowed me to interview them and ask about very private and painful parts of their lives. A number of their partners and husbands also talked with me, and some of their children, too.

Among many scientific books and journal articles used were the following:

Burch, Elizabeth Chamblee. *Mass Tort Deals: Backroom Bargaining in Multidistrict Litigation.* Cambridge, UK: Cambridge University Press, 2019.

Lenzer, Jeanne. *The Danger Within Us: America's Untested, Unregulated Medical Device Industry and One Man's Battle to Survive It.* Boston: Little, Brown and Company, 2017.

Shobeiri, S. Abbas, ed. *The Innovation and Evolution of Medical Devices: Vaginal Mesh Kits.* New York: Springer Publishing, 2018.

Weber, Anne. "Are New Tools for Correcting Prolapse and Incontinence Better Just Because They're New?" *OBG Management* 23, no. 10 (October 2011): e3–e8.

Donohue, Julie. "A History of Drug Advertising: The Evolving Roles of Consumers and Consumer Protection." *Milbank Quarterly: A Multidisciplinary Journal of Population Health and Health Policy* 84, no. 4 (December 2006): 659–99.

Bieman, Jennifer. "London Researchers Examine Psychological Fallout of Incontinence Surgery Complications." *London Free Press* (January 9, 2019).

Heneghan, Carl J., Ben Goldacre, Igho Onakpoya, Jeffrey K. Aronson, Tom Jefferson, Annette Pluddemann, and Kamal R Mahtani. Trials of transvaginal mesh devices for pelvic organ prolapse: A systematic database review of the US FDA approval process. *BMJ Open.* 2017; 7(12): e017125. Published online 2017 Dec. 6. DOI: 10.1136/bmjopen-2017-017125.

Siegal, A. L., et al. High incidence of vaginal mesh extrusion using the intravaginal slingplasty sling. *Journal of Urology.* 2005.

Trabuco, E. C. The Rise and Fall of Mesh in Pelvic Surgery and the Shortcomings of Medical Device Regulation. *Obstetrics & Gynecology.* September 2018.

Ostergard, Donald R. Lessons from the past: Directions for the future. Do new marketed surgical procedures and grafts produce ethical, personal liability, and legal concerns for physicians? *International Urogynecology Journal.* 2007.

Wall, L. Lewis, Douglas Brown. The perils of commercially driven surgical innovation. *Journal of Obstetrics & Gynecology.* 2010.

Kobashi, Kathleen C., Roger Dmochowski, Sharron L. Mee, Jacek Mostwin, Victor W. Nitti, Phillipe E. Zimmern, Gary E. Leach. Erosion of woven polyester pubovaginal sling. *Journal of Urology.* December 1999.

Littman, Paul M., Patrick J. Culligan. The Rapid Evolution of Vaginal Mesh Delivery Systems for the Correction of Pelvic Organ Prolapse: Part I. *Female Patient.* 2009.

Ducey, Ariel. The short lifecycle of a surgical device—Literature analysis using McKinlay's 7-stage model (TVT-Secur). *Health Policy & Technology.* 2015.

Feste, Joseph R., Craig A. Winkel. Is the Standard of Care What We Think It Is? *Journal of the Society of Laparoendoscopic Surgeons.* 1999.

Maher, Christopher. There is still a place for vaginal mesh in urogynaecology. *BJOG Debate.* Published 14 May 2019.

Mowat, Alexandra E., Christopher Maher. Transvaginal mesh: Let's not repeat the mistakes of the past. *Australian and New Zealand Journal of Obstetrics and Gynaecology.* March 2017.

Altman, Daniel, et al. Anterior Colporrhaphy versus Transvaginal Mesh for Pelvic-Organ Prolapse. *New England Journal of Medicine.* May 2011.

Blandon RE, Gebhart JB, Trabuco EC, Klingele CJ. Complications from vaginally placed mesh in pelvic reconstructive surgery. *Int*

Urogynecol J Pelvic Floor Dysfunct. 2009 May;20(5):523-31. 2009 Feb 10. https://www.ncbi.nlm.nih.gov/pubmed/19209374.

Lee D, Dillon B, Lemack G, Gomelsky A, Zimmern P. Transvaginal mesh kits—how "serious" are the complications and are they reversible? *Urology.* 2013 Jan;81(1):43-8. DOI: 10.1016/j.urology .2012.07.098. Epub 2012 Nov 30. https://www.ncbi.nlm.nih.gov /pubmed/23200966.

Woodman, Patrick. "So They've Taken Away My Pelvic Mesh: Now What?" Presentation. Michigan State University. October 2016.

Hota, L. S. TVT-Secur (Hammock) versus TVT-Obturator: A Randomized Trial of Suburethral Sling Operative Procedures. *Female Pelvic Med Reconstructive Surgery.* 2012.

Petros, P. Creating a gold standard surgical device: Scientific discoveries leading to TVT and Beyond—Ulf Ulmsten Memorial Lecture 2014. *International Urogynecology Journal.* 2015.

Togami, Joanna, Elizabeth Brown, J. Christian Winters. Vaginal mesh—The controversy. *F1000 Reports Medicine.* 2012. https:// www.ncbi.nlm.nih.gov/pmc/articles/PMC3506218/.

Maher, Christopher. The way forward after the transvaginal mesh decade. *Obstetrics & Gynaecology.* 28 January 2018. https://doi .org/10.1111/tog.12471.

Maher, Christopher, Nir Haya. The Transvaginal Mesh Decade. *Expert Review of Obstetrics & Gynecology.* 2013 (Vol. 8, Issue 5).

Weber, Anne. ACOG Clinical Practice Bulletin. 2007.

Gornall, Jonathan. The trial that launched millions of mesh implant procedures: Did money compromise the outcome? *British Medical Journal.* October 2018.

Iglesia, Cheryl B. Transvaginal mesh for prolapse: Where are we in 2016? Clinical Review: *OBG Management*. March 2016. https://www.mdedge.com/obgyn/article/107051/gynecology/transvaginal-mesh-prolapse-where-are-we-2016/page/0/1.

Maher, Christopher. Explaining the vaginal mesh controversy. The University of Queensland Australia Faculty of Medicine. 7 June 2017. https://medicine.uq.edu.au/article/2017/06/explaining-vaginal-mesh-controversy.

Gornall, Jonathan. Vaginal mesh implants: Putting the relations between UK doctors and industry in plain sight. BMJ. 2018. DOI: 10.1136/bmj.k4164.

Gornall, Jonathan. How mesh became a four letter word. *BMJ*. 2018. DOI: 10.1136/bmj.k4137.

Allan, Chris, et al. Europe's new device regulations fail to protect the public. *BMJ*. 2018. DOI: 10.1136/bmj.k4205.

Heneghan, Carl, et al. Surgical mesh and patient safety. BMJ (2018). DOI: 10.1136/bmj.k4231.

Abstracts from the Joint Meeting of the International Continence Society and the International Urogynecological Association 34th Annual Meeting. Paris, France, 25–27 August 2004. *Neurourol Urodyn*. 2004;23(5-6):396–610.

Rui Liang, Katrina Knight, Steve Abramowitch, and Pamela A. Moallia. Exploring the basic science of prolapse meshes. *Curr Opin Obstet Gynecol*. 2016. https://www.ncbi.nlm.nih.gov/pmc/articles/PMC5161092/.

Iglesia, Cheryl B., Andrew I. Sokol, Eric R. Sokol, Bela I. Kudish, Robert E. Gutman, Joanna L. Peterson, Susan Shott. Vaginal Mesh for Prolapse: A Randomized Controlled Trial. *Obstetrics*

& Gynecology. August 2010 (Volume 116, Issue 2): pp 293–303.
https://journals.lww.com/greenjournal/Fulltext/2010/08000/Vaginal
_Mesh_for_Prolapse__A_Randomized_Controlled.9.aspx.

Zargar, Nasim, Andrew Carr. The regulatory ancestral network of surgical meshes. University of Oxford, United Kingdom. *PLOS ONE.*
June 19, 2018. https://doi.org/10.1371/journal.pone.0197883.

Talley, Anne D., Bridget R. Rogers, Vladimir Iakovlev, Russell F. Dunn,
Scott A. Guelcher. Oxidation and degradation of polypropylene
transvaginal mesh. *J Biomater Sci Polym Ed.* Published online: 13
Jan 2017. Pp. 444–58.

Wong KS, Nguyen JN, White T, Menefee SA, Walter AJ, Krulewitch
CJ, Anderson-Smits CT, Jakus-Waldman SM. Adverse events
associated with pelvic organ prolapse surgeries that use implants.
Obstet Gynecol. 2013 Dec;122(6):1239–45. DOI: 10.1097
/AOG.0000000000000008.

Heneghan, Carl. TVT: Seventeen-year follow-up and the shrinking
denominator effect. *BMJ EBM.* Posted on 12 September 2018.
https://blogs.bmj.com/bmjebmspotlight/2018/09/12/tvy
-seventeen-year-follow-up-and-the-misleading-effect/.

Surgical Mesh for POP and SUI: 510(k) Not Rigorous Enough.
General Surgery News. February 24, 2016.

TVT-SECUR Expert Report for Ralph Zipper, MD FPMRS Plaintiffs
(Vaginal Mesh). https://www.docketbird.com/court-documents
/USA-vs-See/Exhibit-E/wvsd-2:2012-md-02327-05124-005.

Heneghan, Carl. What a Mesh. *BMJ EBM.* Posted on 4 April 2019.
https://blogs.bmj.com/bmjebmspotlight/2019/04/04/what-a
-mesh/.

Naumann, G., S. Albrich, C. Skala, R. Laterza, H. Kölbl. Single
-Incision Slings (SIS)—A New Option for the Surgical
Treatment of Female Stress Urinary Incontinence. *Geburtshilfe
Frauenheilkd.* 2012. https://www.ncbi.nlm.nih.gov/pmc/articles
/PMC4168529/?report=printable.

Heneghan, Carl J., Ben Goldacre, Igho Onakpoya, Jeffrey K Aronson,
Tom Jefferson, Annette Pluddemann, Kamal R Mahtani. Trials of
transvaginal mesh devices for pelvic organ prolapse: A systematic
database review of the US FDA approval process. *BMJ OPEN.*
November 2017.

Lucente, Vicent R. Laparoscopic Burch colposuspension for stress
urinary incontinence: When, how, and why? *OBG Management.*
2003 February;15(2):20–34.

Highlights from the 2018 Society of Gynecologic Surgeons Scientific
Meeting. May 2, 2018. https://www.mdedge.com/obgyn/article
/162377/gynecology/highlights-2018-society-gynecologic
-surgeons-scientific-meeting.

Rios, A. G., Ephraim, S., Murphy, M., & Lucente, V. A Retrospective Comparison of Dyspareunia and Mesh Exposure Outcomes
for Patients Who Have Undergone Gynemesh (PROLIFT) and
Novasilk (EXAIR) for Treatment of Pelvic Organ Prolapse (POP).
Neurology and Urodynamics. (Vol. 35, pp. S45–S46). (February
2016).

Trabuco, Emmanuel C., Victor M Montori. The Rise and Fall of Mesh
in Pelvic Surgery and the Shortcomings of Medical Device Regulation. *Urogynecology Obstetrics & Gynecology.* September 2018.

J&J Unit Workers Say Biz Knew Pelvic Mesh Device Risks. *Law360.*
29 November 2017. https://www.law360.com/articles/989262
/j-j-unit-workers-say-biz-knew-pelvic-mesh-device-risks.

Pharmaceuticals/Health Products. OpenSecrets.org. 20 June 2019. https://www.opensecrets.org/lobby/indusclient.php?id=H04.

Six "diseases" created by big pharma. *Dr. Micozzi's Insiders' Cures.* 1 October 2015. https://drmicozzi.com/six-diseases-created-by-big-pharma.

A History of Drug Advertising: The Evolving Roles of Consumers and Consumer Protection. NCBI. December 2006. https://www.ncbi.nlm.nih.gov/pmc/articles/PMC2690298/#b4.

Discovery of Polypropylene and the Development of a New High-Density Polyethylene. ACS.org. 12 November 1999. https://www.acs.org/content/dam/acsorg/education/whatischemistry/landmarks/polypropylene/discovery-of-polypropylene-and-development-of-high-density-polyethylene-commemorative-booklet.pdf.

Past, Present and Future of Surgical Meshes: A Review. NCBI. September 2017. https://www.ncbi.nlm.nih.gov/pmc/articles/PMC5618132/.

The trial that launched millions of mesh implant procedures: Did money compromise the outcome? BMJ.com. 10 October 2018. https://www.bmj.com/content/363/bmj.k4155.

Mesh Midurethral Slings for Stress Urinary Incontinence. AUGS. January 2014. https://www.augs.org/assets/1/6/AUGS-SUFU_MUS_Position_Statement.pdf.

The damning vaginal mesh dossier: Shocking failures behind the scandal—and the man who made millions from inventing them. *Daily Mail.* 15 October 2018. https://www.dailymail.co.uk/health/article-6278979/The-damning-vaginal-mesh-dossier-shocking-failures-scandal.html.

How Fen-Phen, a Diet 'Miracle,' Rose and Fell. *New York Times*. 23
    September 1997. https://www.nytimes.com/1997/09/23/science
    /how-fen-phen-a-diet-miracle-rose-and-fell.html.

What have we learned from Vioxx? *BMJ*. 18 January 2007. https://
    www.bmj.com/content/334/7585/120.

Public Law 94-295 94th Congress. Govinfo.gov. 28 May 1976.
    https://www.govinfo.gov/content/pkg/STATUTE-90/pdf
    /STATUTE-90-Pg539.pdf.

"A History of Medical Device Regulation & Oversight in the United
    States." FDA. 8 August 2018. https://www.fda.gov/medical
    -devices/overview-device-regulation/history-medical-device
    -regulation-oversight-united-states.

"Suffering in Silence from a Medical Device—Surgical Mesh (Part 2)."
    Legal Examiner. 8 April 2009. http://news.legalexaminer.com
    /national-news/Suffering-in-Silence-From-A-Medical-Device—
    Surgical-Mesh-Part-2.aspx?googleid=260612#ixzz5rPggdnBP.

"Polypropylene Vaginal Mesh Grafts in Gynecology." ResearchGate.
    October 2010. https://www.researchgate.net/publication
    /46393542_Polypropylene_Vaginal_Mesh_Grafts_in_Gynecology.

"Women vs. Big Pharma in the Battle Over Trans-vaginal Mesh."
    Dallas Observer. 12 September 2014. https://www.dallasobserver
    .com/news/women-vs-big-pharma-in-the-battle-over-trans
    -vaginal-mesh-6433733.

"Single-Incision Sling System." Boston Scientific. 20 June 2019.
    https://www.bostonscientific.com/en-US/products/mid
    -urethral-slings/solyx.html.

"BOSTON SCIENTIFIC CORP., PELVIC REPAIR SYSTEM PROD-
    UCTS LIABILITY LITIGATION PreTrial Order #14." wvsd

.uscourts.gov. 22 August 2012. https://www.wvsd.uscourts.gov
/mdl/boston/pdfs/PTO_14.pdf.

"Lessons from the past: Directions for the future." *International
Urogynecology Journal*. June 2007. https://link.springer.com
/article/10.1007%2Fs00192-007-0330-z.

"Pelvic organ prolapse: Overview." InformedHealth.org. 23 August
2018. https://www.ncbi.nlm.nih.gov/books/NBK525783/.

"Transvaginal mesh: A historical review and update of the current
state of affairs in the United States." *International Urogynecology
Journal*. 22 August 2016. https://www.ncbi.nlm.nih.gov/pubmed
/27549225.

"Surgery for Pelvic Organ Prolapse." ACOG. October 2018. https://
www.acog.org/Patients/FAQs/Surgery-for-Pelvic-Organ
-Prolapse?IsMobileSet=false.

"Gynecological mesh: The medical device that has 100,000 women
suing." *60 Minutes*. 17 April 2019. https://www.cbsnews.com
/news/boston-scientific-gynecological-mesh-the-medical
-device-that-has-100000-women-suing-2019-04-17/.

"Talking about Slings and Meshes. There is a difference!" Central
Florida Urogynecology. Accessed July 30, 2018. http://www
.cfurogyn.com/articles/prolapse/SlingsAndMeshes.html.

"Sling vs. Mesh: What You Need to Know." Urogynecology, University
of Colorado. 9 October 2015. https://urogyn
.coloradowomenshealth.com/blog/sling-vs-mesh.

"Colporrhaphy." *Encyclopedia of Surgery*. Accessed August 6, 2018.
http://www.surgeryencyclopedia.com/Ce-Fi/Colporrhaphy.html.

"Malpractice Premiums and the Supply of Obstetricians." Sagepub. com. Accessed 20 June 2019. https://journals.sagepub.com/doi /pdf/10.5034/inquiryjrnl_47.01.48.

"Revealed: Johnson & Johnson's 'irresponsible' actions over vaginal mesh implant." *Guardian*. 29 September 2017. https://www .theguardian.com/society/2017/sep/29/revealed-johnson -johnsons-irresponsible-actions-over-vaginal-mesh-implant.

"To evaluate the safety and efficacy of the TVT-Secur procedure in the treatment of stress urinary incontinence in women." *Med J Armed Forces India*. January 2017. https://www.ncbi.nlm.nih.gov /pmc/articles/PMC5221397/.

"11 Horror Stories from the Australian Pelvic-Mesh Implant Report." *Women's Health*. 28 March 2018. https://www.womenshealthmag .com/health/a19622268/australian-pelvic-mesh-report-stories/.

"Vaginal mesh has caused health problems in many women, even as some surgeons vouch for its safety and efficacy." *Washington Post*. 20 January 2019. https://www.washingtonpost.com/national /health-science/vaginal-mesh-has-caused-health-problems -in-many-women-even-as-some-surgeons-vouch-for-its-safety -and-efficacy/2019/01/18/1c4a2332-ff0f-11e8-ad40 -cdfd0e0dd65a_story.html?utm_term=.16d4155c9f5b.

"Statement from FDA Commissioner Scott Gottlieb, MD, and Jeff Shuren, MD, Director of the Center for Devices and Radiological Health, on efforts to evaluate materials in medical devices to address potential safety questions." FDA. 15 March 2019. https:// www.fda.gov/news-events/press-announcements/statement -fda-commissioner-scott-gottlieb-md-and-jeff-shuren-md -director-center-devices-and-3?fbclid= IwAR2pylqez4Ez3RRInz48ZR0d0e7m8_e _7WadEku3hJzQEtzBoLX6_pV-now.

"Vaginal mesh left me in agony. When will women's health be taken seriously?" *Guardian.* 27 April 2017. https://www.theguardian .com/commentisfree/2017/apr/27/vaginal-mesh-women-health -bladders-bowels-sex-lives-nhs-operations.

"Here Are the Most Heartbreaking Letters to an Inquiry on Mesh Implants." BuzzFeed.News. 7 September 2017. https://www .buzzfeed.com/ginarushton/here-are-the-most-heartbreaking -letters-to-mesh-inquiry.

"Failed vaginal mesh implants for stress incontinence boost depression risk, study says." *Star.* 9 January 2019. https://www.thestar .com/news/canada/2019/01/09/failed-vaginal-mesh-implants -for-stress-incontinence-boost-depression-risk-study-says.html.

"How Doctors Take Women's Pain Less Seriously." *Atlantic.* 15 October 2015. https://www.theatlantic.com/health/archive/2015/10 /emergency-room-wait-times-sexism/410515/.

"Preventing Sexual Violence." CDC. Accessed June 20, 2019. https:// www.cdc.gov/violenceprevention/sexualviolence/fastfact .html?CDC_AA_refVal=https%3A%2F%2Fwww.cdc.gov%2F violenceprevention%2Fsexualviolence%2Fdefinitions.html.

"Not All Doctors Get Informed Consent—Here's Why It's Hurting Patients." *Forbes.* 28 March 2016. https://www.forbes.com/sites /amino/2016/03/28/not-all-doctors-get-informed-consent-heres -why-its-hurting-patients/#882f71d496c6.

"Australia investigates implants that left some women with 'rotting pelvises.'" CNN. 29 March 2018. https://www.cnn.com/2018/03 /28/health/pelvic-mesh-implant-australia-senate-intl/index.html.

"National Implant Registries." Kaiser Permanente. Accessed June 20, 2019. https://national-implantregistries.kaiserpermanente.org /about.

"Trial Lawyers' Tricks Put Women's Health at Risk." Morning Consult. 27 February 2019. https://morningconsult.com/opinions/trial-lawyers-tricks-put-womens-health-at-risk/.

"Transvaginal Mesh Kits—How 'Serious' Are the Complications and Are They Reversible?" Science Direct. January 2013. https://www.sciencedirect.com/science/article/pii/S009042951201076X.

"Get the facts about transvaginal mesh complications." Mayo Clinic. Accessed April 19, 2018. https://www.mayoclinic.org/diseases-conditions/pelvic-organ-prolapse/in-depth/transvaginal-mesh-complications/art-20110300?pg=2.

"Surgery Under Scrutiny: What Went Wrong with Vaginal Mesh." WBUR. 4 November 2011. http://commonhealth.legacy.wbur.org/2011/11/surgery-under-scrutiny-what-went-wrong-with-vaginal-mesh.

"FDA strengthens requirements for surgical mesh for the transvaginal repair of pelvic organ prolapse to address safety risks." FDA. Accessed April 24, 2018, https://www.fda.gov/NewsEvents/Newsroom/PressAnnouncements/ucm479732.htm.

"Transvaginal Mesh Removal." UCLA Health. Accessed April 24, 2018. http://obgyn.ucla.edu/mesh-related-complications.

"Removal of Faulty Mesh for Incontinence." WebMD. Accessed April 24, 2018. https://www.webmd.com/urinary-incontinence-oab/news/20140519/removal-of-faulty-mesh-for-incontinence-may-not-improve-womens-symptoms#1.

"Women come from across world to have St. Louis doctor remove their pelvic mesh." *St. Louis Post Dispatch*. 15 November 2014. https://www.stltoday.com/lifestyles/health-med-fit/health/women-come-from-across-world-to-have-st-louis-doctor/article_0deb184e-007a-543c-8cd4-884620c1263d.html.

"Complications from transvaginal pubovaginal slings using bone anchor fixation." NCBI. December 2004. https://www.ncbi.nlm .nih.gov/pubmed/15596184.

"'Scandal' of vaginal mesh removal rates revealed by NHS records." *Guardian*. 15 August 2017. https://www.theguardian.com /society/2017/aug/15/scandal-of-vaginal-mesh-removal-rates -revealed-by-nhs-records.

"Urogynecologic Surgical Mesh: Update on the Safety and Effectiveness of Transvaginal Placement for Pelvic Organ Prolapse." FDA. July 2001. https://www.fda.gov/media/81123/download.

"New Zealand becomes first country to fully ban controversial vaginal mesh procedures." *Independent.* 12 December 2017. https://www .independent.co.uk/news/world/australasia/vaginal-tvt-mesh -scandal-incontinence-prolapse-ban-suspension-new-zealand -australia-nice-guidelines-a8105861.html.

"Surgical Mesh Implants." MedSafe. 31 January 2018. https://medsafe .govt.nz/hot/alerts/UrogynaecologicaSurgicalMeshImplants.asp.

"Number of women in Australia who have had transvaginal mesh implants and related matters." Parliament of Australia. 28 March 2018. https://www.aph.gov.au/Parliamentary_Business /Committees/Senate/Community_Affairs/MeshImplants/Report.

"Use of transvaginal mesh devices put on pause, says Minister for Health." *Irish Times*. 24 July 2018. https://www.irishtimes.com /news/health/use-of-transvaginal-mesh-devices-put-on -pause-says-minister -for-health-1.3575463.

"FDA takes action to protect women's health, orders manufacturers of surgical mesh intended for transvaginal repair of pelvic organ prolapse to stop selling all devices." FDA. 16 April 2019. https://

www.fda.gov/news-events/press-announcements/fda-takes
-action-protect-womens-health-orders-manufacturers
-surgical-mesh-intended-transvaginal.

"Reclassification of Urogynecologic Surgical Mesh Implementation."
FDA. 26 February 2016. https://www.fda.gov/media/96464
/download.

"Scottish government offers formal apology to mesh victims." *Daily
Mail*. 25 October 2018. https://www.dailymail.co.uk/wires/pa
/article-6316221/Scottish-Government-offers-formal-apology
-mesh-victims.html?fbclid=IwAR273Bwd3XJcX2
-DE8Nwh9flCt27sSXAD2MbeuJAIfzuCCrVAEqM1C0IAGI.

"Pelvic mesh: Obstetrician says profession must learn from scandal,
calls for register." ABC News Australia. 23 October 2018. https://
www.abc.net.au/news/2018-10-24/medical-profession-must
-learn-from-pelvic-mesh-mistakes-doctor/10419242.

"Mesh implants: Government issues national apology over 'agony and
pain' caused by device." ABC News Australia. 9 October 2018.
https://www.abc.net.au/news/2018-10-10/mesh-implants
-government-issues-apology-to-women/10355546.

"Pelvic mesh implants: How tracking vehicle parts is easier than
medical devices." ABC News Australia. 26 March 2018. https://
www.abc.net.au/news/2018-03-27/pelvic-mesh-implants
-tracking-medical-devices/9588070.

"TGA actions after review into urogynaecological surgical mesh
implants." Australian Department of Health. 17 May 2019.
https://www.tga.gov.au/alert/tga-actions-after-review
-urogynaecological-surgical-mesh-implants.

"Vaginal mesh implants: Australia apologises for 'decades of pain.'" BBC. 10 October 2018. https://www.bbc.com/news/world-australia-45806324.

"Mesh Removal in Australia." Australian Department of Health. Accessed 20 June 2019. https://www.ranzcog.edu.au/RANZCOG_SITE/media/RANZCOG-MEDIA/Media%20Centre/Mesh-removal-in-Australia.pdf.

"High Incidence of Vaginal Mesh Extrusion Using the Intravaginal Slingplasty Sling." *Journal of Urology.* October 2005. https://www.sciencedirect.com/science/article/pii/S0022534701686142.

"The perils of commercially driven surgical innovation." *American Journal of Obstetrics and Gynecology.* January 2010. https://www.sciencedirect.com/science/article/pii/S0002937809005390.

"Erosion of Woven Polyester Pubovaginaerosion of Woven Polyester Pubovaginal Sling." *Journal of Urology.* 1 December 1999. https://www.auajournals.org/article/S0022-5347(05)68103-7/references.

"Is the Standard of Care What We Think It Is?" *Journal of the Society of Laparoendoscopic Surgeons.* November 1998. https://www.researchgate.net/publication/12621687_Is_the_Standard_of_Care_What_We_Think_It_Is.

"Transvaginal Mesh Kits—How 'Serious' Are the Complications and Are They Reversible?" *Urology.* January 2013. https://www.sciencedirect.com/science/article/pii/S009042951201076X.

"TVT-Secur (Hammock) Versus TVT-Obturator: A Randomized Trial of Suburethral Sling Operative Procedures." NCBI. 16 July 2013. https://www.ncbi.nlm.nih.gov/pmc/articles/PMC3712515/.

"Creating a gold standard surgical device: Scientific discoveries leading to TVT and beyond." *International Urogynecology Journal.*

19 February 2015. https://link.springer.com/article/10.1007%
2Fs00192-015-2639-3.

"Vaginal mesh—the controversy." NCBI. 1 November 2012. https://
www.ncbi.nlm.nih.gov/pmc/articles/PMC3506218/.

"The trial that launched millions of mesh implant procedures: Did
money compromise the outcome?" *BMJ.* 10 October 2018.
https://www.bmj.com/content/363/bmj.k4155.

"Vaginal mesh implants: Putting the relations between UK doctors
and industry in plain sight." *BMJ.* 10 October 2018. https://www
.bmj.com/content/363/bmj.k4164.

"How mesh became a four-letter word." *BMJ.* 10 October 2018.
https://www.bmj.com/content/363/bmj.k4137.

"Exploring the basic science of prolapse meshes." NCBI. 16 December
2016. https://www.ncbi.nlm.nih.gov/pmc/articles/PMC5161092/.

"Vaginal Mesh for Prolapse: A Randomized Controlled Trial."
The American College of Obstetricians and Gynecologists.
August 2010. https://journals.lww.com/greenjournal
/Fulltext/2010/08000/Vaginal_Mesh_for_Prolapse__A
_Randomized_Controlled.9.aspx.

"The regulatory ancestral network of surgical meshes." University
of Oxford. 19 June 2018. https://www.ndorms.ox.ac.uk
/publications/856881.

"Oxidation and degradation of polypropylene transvaginal mesh."
Journal of Biomaterials Science, Polymer Edition. 11 November
2016. https://www.tandfonline.com/doi/full/10.1080/09205063
.2017.1279045.

"TVT: Seventeen-year follow-up and the shrinking denominator effect." *BMJ Blog.* 12 September 2018. https://blogs.bmj.com /bmjebmspotlight/2018/09/12/tvy-seventeen-year-follow-up -and-the-misleading-effect/.

"What a Mesh." *BMJ Blog.* 4 April 2019. https://blogs.bmj.com /bmjebmspotlight/2019/04/04/what-a-mesh/.

"Single-Incision Slings (SIS)—A New Option for the Surgical Treat-ment of Female Stress Urinary Incontinence." *Geburtshilfe Frauenheilkd.* 23 October 2011. https://www.ncbi.nlm.nih.gov /pmc/articles/PMC4168529/?report=printable.

"Trials of transvaginal mesh devices for pelvic organ prolapse: A sys-tematic database review of the US FDA approval process." *BMJ.* Accessed June 20, 2019. https://bmjopen.bmj.com/content/7/12 /e017125.

"Laparoscopic Burch colposuspension for stress urinary incontinence: When, how, and why?" MDedge. 15 February 2015. https://www .mdedge.com/obgyn/article/61309/laparoscopic-burch -colposuspension-stress-urinary-incontinence -when-how-and-why.

"Highlights from the 2018 Society of Gynecologic Surgeons Scientific Meeting." MDedge. 2 May 2018. https://www.mdedge.com/obgyn /article/162377/gynecology/highlights-2018-society-gynecologic -surgeons-scientific-meeting.

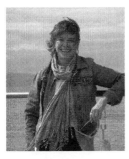

Alicia Mundy is an award-winning author, reporter, and columnist based in Washington, DC. She has covered the health-care and pharmaceutical/medical device industries for 20 years. She focused on Congress and the lobbying of powerful corporations and interest groups representing health-care companies, such as vaginal mesh makers. Her first book, *Dispensing with the Truth*, revealed company secrets about the fen-phen diet-drug scandal and was a semifinalist for the Robert F. Kennedy Book Award. She was a reporter in the DC bureau of the *Wall Street Journal* and later was chief investigator for the Democrats on the Senate Committee on the Budget, looking at the high costs of medicine.

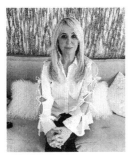

Jennifer Banmiller has been involved in the consumer marketing and media business for 30 years. She is the founder of Wingtip Communications, Inc. and legal consumer advocacy sites such as www.periscopegroup.com. The author of "Salesmanship 101" for attorneys, she is a fervent advocate for consumers in the health-care field.

Made in the
USA
Middletown, DE